Neuroradiology

Neuroradiology
A Case-Based Guide

Swati Goyal

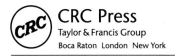

CRC Press
Taylor & Francis Group
Boca Raton London New York

CRC Press is an imprint of the
Taylor & Francis Group, an **informa** business

First edition published 2021
by CRC Press
6000 Broken Sound Parkway NW, Suite 300, Boca Raton, FL 33487-2742

and by CRC Press
2 Park Square, Milton Park, Abingdon, Oxon, OX14 4RN

Library of Congress Cataloging-in-Publication Data
Names: Goyal, Swati, author. Title: Neuroradiology : a case-based guide / by Dr. Swati Goyal. Description: First edition. | Boca Raton, FL : CRC Press, 2020. | Includes bibliographical references and index. | Summary: "This book covers the complete gamut of cases, CT physics, normal anatomy, pitfalls, artefacts, across brain and spine in a single volume with its pragmatic approach. Provides brief description of CT/MR physics, MR sequences, recent advances and neuroradiology interventions"-- Provided by publisher.
Identifiers: LCCN 2020032736 (print) | LCCN 2020032737 (ebook) | ISBN 9780367548001 (hardback) | ISBN 9780367903190 (paperback) | ISBN 9780367903206 (ebook)
Subjects: MESH: Central Nervous System Diseases--diagnostic imaging | Neuroradiography--methods | Case Reports
Classification: LCC RC348 (print) | LCC RC348 (ebook) | NLM WL 141.5.N47 | DDC 616.8/0475--dc23
LC record available at https://lccn.loc.gov/2020032736
LC ebook record available at https://lccn.loc.gov/2020032737

ISBN: 9780367548001 (hbk)
ISBN: 9780367903190 (pbk)
ISBN: 9780367903206 (ebk)

Typeset in Minion
by Deanta Global Publishing Services, Chennai, India

Dedicated to my adorable kids, Prisha and Rushank, who energized me in spite of all the time the task of book writing took me away from them.

Contents

PART III: THE HEAD AND NECK

Preface

Since their genesis in the early 1970s, CT and MRI have engendered colossal ascendancy in diagnostic imaging and have evolved as the cornerstone of medical imaging. In the fullness of time, advances in both their hardware and software have taken place, and these technological upswings have paved the way for innovative and diverse uses of CT/MRI.

As we broaden our horizons in the arena of CT/MRI applications, so must the skills and knowledge of scientists and technologists occupied in this field be developed and expanded.

This book is formulated as a concise teaching guide for the core examination, Neuroradiology, neurology for radiology residents, for general practitioners, and for CT and MRI technicians. Whereas the book has been drafted primarily for trainee radiologists, neurophysicians, neurosurgeons, and CT/MRI technicians, the text, along with the annotated images, will also be valuable to other, more general physicians, such as ophthalmologists and otolaryngorhinologists, interested in medical imaging.

This book is organized into three parts and 16 thematic chapters. Part I constitutes cases of the brain and includes both normal and abnormal findings, with differential diagnosis and relevant images of conditions usually encountered during routine practice, covering each of the pivotal aspects in different chapters. Topics like normal brain development and congenital malformations, normal vascular anatomy and its anomalies, intracranial hemorrhage, trauma, neoplasms, infections, disorders involving white and gray matter, normal CSF circulation and its disorders, phakomatoses, cranial nerves, and the craniovertebral junction have been described in detail.

Part II elucidates the normal anatomy of the spine, various congenital and acquired spinal disorders, and supporting case studies.

Part III includes a brief description of case studies of the head and neck region, separated into eye/orbit, ear, nose, paranasal sinuses, and neck region.

The last chapter incorporates miscellaneous topics, like epilepsy, empty sella, and the current and future role of artificial intelligence (AI) in neuroradiology.

Neuroradiology, in itself, is a comprehensive sub-specialty of radiology, with an endless list of cases and patients presenting in a myriad of ways. This book offers carefully selected case studies, with a concise account of 154 routinely experienced pathologies, illustrated by suitable images. The cases are structured into thematic chapters, to provide an integrated approach for basic learning. Each case study has been drafted logically, commencing with a brief clinical history, relevant imaging findings, and discussion, including differential diagnosis and management, and with suggested readings provided for each chapter.

Appropriate training and expertise are required, along with theoretical knowledge of cases for reporting. The book is an invaluable adjunct to standard textbooks, but is not intended to substitute for them. The book focuses on step-by-step descriptions of cases routinely encountered in neuroradiological imaging, providing support and help in taking certificate examinations, such as the core examination of Neuroradiology, RITE (Residency In-service Training Examination) of the American Academy of Neurology, Neuroradiology CAQ (Certificate of Additional Qualification) examination, ARRT (American Registry of Radiology Technicians), BSc (Bachelor of Science) in medical imaging, and ARMRIT (American Registry of Magnetic Resonance Imaging Technologists).

Bolstered by nearly 400 high-resolution images, obtained with state-of-the-art scanning technology, this essential enchiridion is designed to train the reader how to interpret both CT and MRI images of the brain, spine, head, and neck. It includes valuable background material as case studies, commonly encountered in clinical practice, with reference to normal anatomy, preparing the reader for the challenges of the clinical setting. It can also be used as a readily accessible reference book for use in the midst of a busy clinical day.

This book aims to provide a consolidated resource for the technologists to acquire the knowledge necessary for excellent patient care in the field of neuroradiology.

Acknowledgments

Having an idea and then converting it into a book is as arduous as it sounds; the experience is both challenging and gratifying. I would wholeheartedly like to thank the individuals who helped make this book happen.

I am eternally grateful to my parents, Mrs Poonam Gupta and Dr Ramesh K. Gupta, who taught me the value of education and hard work, and so much more, that has helped me succeed in life.

Writing a second technical book was harder than I thought, but also more rewarding than I could have imagined. None of this would have been possible without my husband Dr Sanjay Goyal, MD Pediatrics, IAS, MPH (JHU), who has stood beside me throughout my career and has been there every step of the way to help me in this phenomenal achievement.

Hearty thanks are owed to my in-laws for their constant emotional support and motivation.

I also offer my sincere gratitude to Professor Bisen, (retired) V.C. Jiwaji University – a visionary academician – for guiding me in the right direction.

I owe a debt of gratitude to my teachers, Dr O.P. Tiwari and Dr Rajesh Malik, who inspired and continue to inspire me to pursue a career in academia.

A task of this size could not be completed without the unwavering support provided by our head of department, Dr Lovely Kaushal. Many thanks are due for her academic vision and positive influences.

Blessed are those who have amazing seniors, who guide and encourage their junior colleagues. I am lucky to have such amazing people in my life. I offer my overwhelming thankfulness to Dr M.K. Mittal, Dr R.P. Kaushal, and Dr Prateek S. Gehlot for magnanimously providing me with images for this book, and for their professional guidance and support.

Wholehearted thanks are due to Dr Sahil Gupta, Dr Shimanku Maheshwari, Dr Parminder Chawla, and Dr. Bhavna Seth (JHU) for their enthusiastic support during this venture.

I would also like to extend my profound personal thanks to my senior colleagues, Dr Vijay Verma, Dr Poornima Maravi, Dr Pinky Patil, and Dr Vivek Soni, for the generous guidance they offered.

Many thanks to my postgraduate students, Dr Sandeep Chauhan (JR-3), Dr Satish (JR-2), and Dr Vignesh (JR-1), for their technical assistance.

I would like to acknowledge and show my appreciation for all the authors and editors, whose books, journals, and websites I have accessed since my medical residency days, without which this book would never have come to fruition.

Immense thanks are due to Miranda Bromage, Publisher; Shivangi Pramanik, Commissioning Editor – Medical; and her editorial assistant, Himani Dwivedi, who green-lighted this book and remained patient throughout the long process. Earnest thanks are also due to the skilled editing and designing teams.

It is indeed a pleasure to express my sincere thanks to those whose time and efforts have helped tremendously in constructing a compilation of this breadth, contributing to the academic richness of this monograph. The list is long, and words are insufficient to convey my heartfelt thanks to the following for their generous gifts of images, line diagrams, and case studies used in this book.

Mahesh K. Mittal, MBBS, MD
Professor, Radiodiagnosis
VM Medical College and Safdarjung Hospital
New Delhi, India
(50 images)

Mukul Sinha, MBBS, MD
Consultant Radio Diagnosis
VM Medical College and Safdarjung Hospital
New Delhi, India
(50 images)

Lovely Kaushal, MBBS, MD
Professor and HoD
Radiodiagnosis
Government Medical College & Hamidia Hospital
Bhopal, India
(75 images)

Prateek S. Gehlot, MBBS, MD
Associate Professor
Radiodiagnosis
R.D. Gardi Medical College and C.R.Gardi
    Hospital
Ujjain (MP), India
(60 images)

Abhishek Prasad, MD
Senior Consultant Radiologist
Fortis Hospital
Mohali, India
(10 images)

Sapna Somani, MD
Senior Consultant Radiologist
Saksham Diagnostic Centre
Gwalior, India
(5 images)

Chandraprakash Ahirwar, MD
Consultant Radiologist
Saral Diagnostic Centre
Bhopal, India
(3 images)

Ratnesh Jain, MBBS, MD
Assistant Professor
Radiodiagnosis
GRMC
Gwalior (MP), India
(10 line diagrams)

Poornima Maravi, MBBS, MD
Associate Professor
Radiodiagnosis
GMCH
Bhopal, India
(4 images)

Sana Mirchia Varma, MBBS, MD
Consultant Radiologist
Mirchia's Diagnostic Centre
Chandigarh, India
(10 case studies)

Sandeep Awal, MBBS, MD, DNB
Consultant Radiologist
Brahmananda Narayana Multispeciality Hospital
(Narayana Health)
Jamshedpur, India
(54 images and 6 case studies)

Jyoti Chaudhary, MBBS, MD
Assistant Professor
Radiodiagnosis
Shri Shankaracharya Institute of Medical Sciences
Bhilai, India
(6 images and 9 case studies)

Saumya Mishra, MBBS, MD
Consultant Radiologist
Asian Institute of Medical Sciences
Dombivli, India
(4 images and 1 case study)

Shweta Thakur, MBBS, MD
Senior Resident
RML Hospital
New Delhi, India
(8 case studies)

Bhagyashree Rathore, MBBS, MD
Senior Resident
Department of Radiodiagnosis
MGM Medical College
Indore, India
(70 images and 10 case studies)

Pooja Rajput, JR-3
GMCH
Bhopal, India
(5 case studies)

Vetrivel K.S.
Junior Resident 1st year
GMCH
Bhopal, India
(1 case study)

Rushank Goyal
CEO
Betsos
Bhopal, India
(AI in Neuroradiology)

About the Author

Swati Goyal, DMRD, DNB, is an Associate Professor in the Department of Radiodiagnosis, the Government Medical College (GMC) and Hospital, Bhopal, India. She is also the author of an international book on abdomino-pelvic sonography for practitioners. Dr Goyal is currently pursuing her PhD in medical sciences. Her various peer-reviewed research papers have been published in both national and international journals. Dr Goyal received her MBBS degree from GMC, Amritsar. After completing her residency from GMC and the Maharaja Yashwant-Rao Hospital (MYH), Indore, she underwent further training in Bhopal, where she was awarded a DNB degree by NBE (National Board of Examinations), in Delhi. Dr Goyal has served as a Senior Resident in Chirayu Medical College, Bhopal, and in the All-India Institute of Medical Sciences Bhopal, before joining GMC Bhopal as an Assistant Professor. She is a life member of the Indian Radiological and Imaging Association. In addition to writing two technical academic books, Dr Goyal is also the author of a non-academic book aimed at the general public, addressing public health issues pertaining to lifestyle ailments, *What a Non-Medico Must Know – The Quintessential Guide to Family Health and Wellness*. Dr Goyal also contributes medical articles for the eminent newspaper, the Times of India, and regularly writes articles pertaining to the medical field on her Facebook page.

Abbreviations

ACA	Anterior Cerebral Artery	**ICP**	Intracranial Pressure
AComA	Anterior Communicating Artery	**MCA**	Middle Cerebral Artery
ADC	Apparent Diffusion Coefficient	**MRI**	Magnetic Resonance Imaging
AI	Artificial Intelligence	**MRS**	Magnetic Resonance Spectroscopy
CECT	Contrast-Enhanced CT	**MTR**	Magnetization Transfer Ratio
CSF	Cerebrospinal Fluid	**NAA**	N-Acetyl Acetate
CNS	Central Nervous System	**PCA**	Posterior Cerebral Artery
CPA	Cerebellopontine Angle	**PComA**	Posterior Communicating Artery
CT	Computed Tomography	**Pt**	Patient
DDs	Differential Diagnoses	**SIFT**	Scale-Invariant Feature Transform
DSA	Digital Subtraction Angiography	**STIR**	Short Tau Inversion Recovery
DTI	Diffusion Tensor Imaging	**SURF**	Speeded-Up Robust Features
DWI	Diffusion Weighted Imaging	**SWI**	Susceptibility Weighted Imaging
FLAIR	Fluid Attenuation Inversion Recovery	**T1WI**	T1-Weighted Imaging
GRE	Gradient Echo Sequence	**T2WI**	T2-Weighted Imaging
GWM	Gray–White Matter	**USG**	Ultrasonography
ICA	Internal Carotid Artery		

Normal Brain Development and Congenital Malformations

Normal brain development has four phases:

1) *Dorsal induction* involves the process of neurulation or neural tube formation.

   The appearance of the *neural plate* (at around 4.5–5 weeks of gestation), followed by its invagination, leads to the formation of a *neural groove*. Thickening and proliferation of the lateral portion of the groove form *neural folds*. The apposition of the neural folds in the midline forms the *neural tube*.

   Malformations at dorsal induction include anencephaly, cephalocele, and Chiari 2 malformation.

   Secondary neurulation involves the formation of the distal spine, including the skull, dura, pia, and vertebrae, at 4–5 weeks. Abnormalities at this phase result in spinal dysraphic disorders like spina bifida occulta, meningocele, lipomeningocele, neurenteric cysts, dermal sinus, caudal regression syndrome, etc., which will be discussed in the next section.

2) *Ventral induction* involves formation of primary brain vesicles by rostral expansion of the neural tube. The proximal two-thirds of the neural tube develops into the future brain, with the caudal one-third developing into the future spinal cord. The lumen of the tube develops into the ventricular system of the brain and the central canal of the spinal cord.

   Abnormal development at this time results in anomalies such as holoprosencephaly, hydrocephalus, aqueductal stenosis, corpus callosum agenesis, and posterior fossa malformations such as the Dandy-Walker malformation, cerebellar hypoplasia, and rhombencephalosynapsis.

3) *Neuronal proliferation, differentiation, migration, and histogenesis* occur at around 8–22 weeks of gestation. At this time, neurons migrate peripherally from the germinal matrix (that lines the ventricular surface) to the pia mater/cortex. Brain insults during this time result in abnormalities like lissencephaly (smooth brain) to schizencephaly (split brain), polymicrogyria, laminar/focal heterotopia, microcephaly, megalencephaly, focal cortical dysplasia, hemimegalencephaly, schizencephaly, vascular anomalies, and phakomatoses.

4) *Myelination* will be discussed in Chapter 6.

CASE STUDIES

Chiari Malformations

Disorder of primary neurulation.

CLINICAL

Headache, vertigo, sensory changes, limb weakness, ataxia.

IMAGING

Chiari 0 Malformation

Syrinx without tonsillar ectopia.

Chiari 1 Malformation

Congenital tonsillar ectopia with inferior displacement/herniation (>5 mm) of elongated and pointed tonsils into the upper cervical canal

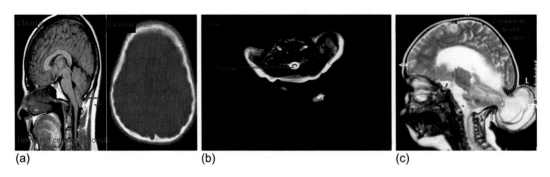

Figure 1.1 (a and b) Chiari 2 malformation, (c) Chiari 3 malformation.

through the foramen magnum. It is associated with:

- Syringohydromyelia (syrinx) – CSF accumulation within the spinal cord
- Hydrocephalus
- Osseous anomalies like basilar invagination, atlanto-occipital assimilation, platybasia, and Klippel-Feil syndrome

Chiari 1.5 Malformation

Inferior displacement of the cerebellar tonsils and brainstem.

Chiari 2 Malformation

- Hydrocephalus
  - Lateral ventricles – colpocephaly
  - 3rd ventricle – large massa intermedia
  - 4th ventricle – tube-like, elongated, and inferiorly displaced
- Brain parenchyma
  - Hypoplastic fenestrated falx with interdigitating gyri (serrated interhemispheric fissure)
  - Beaked tectum
  - Medullary spur and kink
  - Inferiorly displaced vermis
  - May be associated with dysgenetic corpus callosum, polymicrogyria, heterotopias
- Skull and dura
  - Lacunar skull
  - Small posterior fossa with low-lying transverse sinuses and torcular Herophili
  - Gaping foramen magnum
  - Concave petrous ridges and clivus
  - Heart-shaped tentorial incisura
  - Upwardly herniating cerebellum, engulfing the brainstem (towering cerebellum)
- Spinal cord

- Myelomeningocele
- Syrinx
- Retroflexed odontoid with crowded foramen magnum
- Diastematomyelia and segmentation anomalies

Chiari 3 Malformation

- Chiari 2 malformation + encephalocele (low occipital/high cervical)
- Skull defect with herniation of intracranial contents like cerebellum and occipital lobes

Chiari 4 Malformation

- Cerebellar hypo/aplasia
- CSF-filled posterior fossa
- Small brainstem (small and flattened pons)
- No hydrocephalus and myelomeningocele

DDs OF TONSILLAR HERNIATION

Differential diagnoses due to reduced CSF pressure and raised intracranial pressure.

- An ancillary sign of an intracranial mass effect like a tumor, hemorrhage, trauma, etc., leading to the inferior displacement of posterior cranial fossa structures.
- Bony abnormalities that reduce posterior fossa volume, e.g., craniosynostosis, achondroplasia, acromegaly, osteogenesis imperfecta, Paget's disease, etc.
- Intracranial hypotension (CSF hypovolemia) – CSF leakage that may be idiopathic, iatrogenic (lumbar puncture, spinal surgery), presenting with postural headaches, vomiting, etc. It is associated with subdural collections, dural venous sinus distension, and pachymeningeal (dural) enhancement.

- Intracranial hypertension (pseudotumor cerebri) is also associated with empty sella, prominent and tortuous optic nerve sheath, dural venous thrombosis, etc. Meningoceles with secondary CSF leak can present with intracranial hypotension.

MANAGEMENT

Surgery and symptomatic management.

Lissencephaly

Defect in the cortical organization or neuronal migration results in a smooth brain, with a paucity of sulcal and gyral development.

CLINICAL

Microcephaly, seizures, developmental delays, failure to thrive.

IMAGING

See Table 1.1.

MANAGEMENT

Thorough genetic evaluation.

Gray Matter Heterotopias

Malformations of cortical development caused by a defect in neuronal migration. It can be present anywhere from the walls of the lateral ventricles to subcortical locations.

CLINICAL

Seizures, delayed milestones.

IMAGING

Heterotopic gray matter exhibits the signal intensity of normal gray matter; does not enhance or calcify (Figure 1.2).

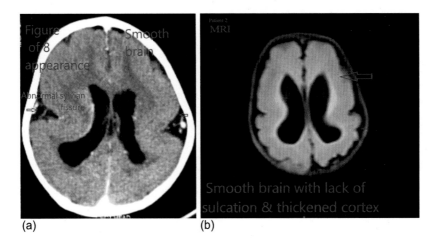

(a)   (b)

Figure 1.2 (a and b) Smooth brain (lissencephaly).

Table 1.1 Imaging Findings of Three Types of Lissencephaly

Type 1	Type 2	Type 3
• Colpocephaly • Smooth gray–white matter interface • Thickened cortex with broad, flat gyri • Shallow Sylvian fissure ("figure of 8") • Subcortical heterotopias • Parenchymal calcifications (if due to intrauterine infections) • Miller-Dieker syndrome – microphthalmia with retinal detachment	• Thickened cortex with polymicrogyria • Cobblestone nodularity • Hypomyelination of underlying white matter • Hydrocephalus • Walker-Warburg syndrome	• Microcephaly • Moderately thickened cortex • Hydrocephalus • Hypoplastic cerebellum and brainstem

Gray matter heterotopias can be broadly divided into:

Subependymal nodular heterotopias
- The gray matter nodules appear in varying sizes to line the germinal matrix walls of the lateral ventricles, with the nodules projecting inward
- It usually shows normal gyral and sulcal patterns

Band/laminar heterotopias (Figure 1.3a)
- Smoothly marginated, symmetrical bands of gray matter interspersed in normal white matter between the cortex and ventricular walls (double cortex)
- It is included in the lissencephaly spectrum

Subcortical heterotopias (Figure 1.3b)
- Curvilinear heterotopias – the gray matter shows continuity to the overlying cortex, which may be thinned out
- Nodular subcortical heterotopias have no such communication

DDs
- Subependymal nodules of tuberous sclerosis show calcification
- Schizencephaly (closed-lip) – outward pouching of the lateral ventricles

ANCILLARY
They may be associated with ventriculomegaly, callosal abnormalities, cortical dysplasias, and small ipsilateral cerebral hemispheres.

Schizencephaly (Split Brain)

Injury to the germinal matrix during the early stage of gestation results in loss of full thickness of the cerebral tissue and eventually a CSF-filled cleft forms, extending from the ependymal surface to the pia mater through the white matter. It can be unilateral or bilateral.

Types:

- *Closed-lip* – closely apposed lips and nipple-like outpouching at the ependymal surface
- *Open-lip* – widely separated cleft lips filled with CSF, with severe clinical manifestations

CLINICAL
Seizures, mental retardation, and developmental or motor delays.

IMAGING
CT and MRI:

- Gray matter-lined CSF-filled cleft that connects the subarachnoid space to the lateral ventricles
- Polymicrogyria, hydrocephalus, corpus callosum abnormalities, heterotopias, and absence of cavum septum pellucidum

DDs
- Porencephalic cyst – white matter-lined, usually follows an event of encephalomalacia
- Focal cortical dysplasia – cleft does not extend up to the ventricular surface

MANAGEMENT
Medical and physical therapy.

Holoprosencephaly

Spectrum of disorders that occurs due to failure or defect in the cleavage. It encompasses various

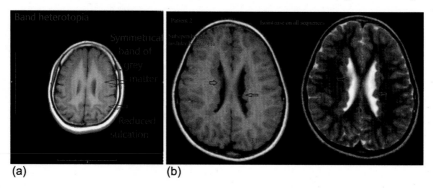

(a)   (b)

Figure 1.3 (a) Band heterotopia, (b) subependymal nodular heterotopia.

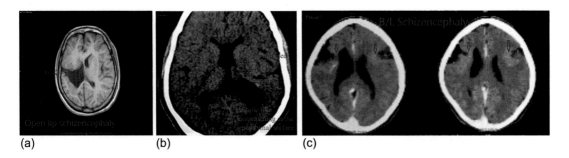

Figure 1.4 (a) Open-lip schizencephaly, (b) closed-lip schizencephaly, (c) bilateral schizencephaly.

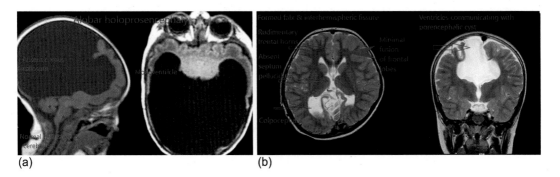

Figure 1.5 (a) Alobar holoprosencephaly, (b) lobar holoprosencephaly, colpocephaly with a porencephalic cyst.

Table 1.2 Differentiation between Three Types of Holoprosencephaly

	Alobar	Semilobar	Lobar
Ventricle	Monoventricle	Rudimentary temporal horns	Rudimentary frontal horns
Basal ganglia, thalamus	Fused	May be partially fused	Separate
Falx/ interhemispheric fissure	Absent, with pancake configuration of brain Normal cerebellum and brainstem	Partial, with fusion of more than 50% of frontal lobe	Present
Corpus callosum	Absent	Splenium may be seen	Present except genu and rostrum
DDs	Hydranencephaly Severe hydrocephalus	Porencephaly Arachnoid cyst	Septo-optic dysplasia(well-formed frontal horns, with hypoplastic optic nerves)

forms ranging from alobar, semilobar, and lobar types, in order of decreasing severity.

CLINICAL

Abnormal facies, cyclopia, endocrinopathies, and mental retardation.

IMAGING

- Absent cavum septum pellucidum (see Table 1.2)

MANAGEMENT

Accurate prenatal diagnosis and counseling.

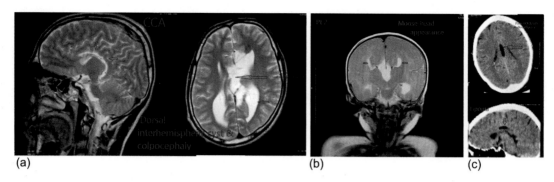

Figure 1.6 (a) Corpus callosum agenesis with associated dorsal interhemispheric cyst, (b) "moose-head" appearance, (c) partial callosal agenesis with callosal lipoma.

ANCILLARY

- *Middle interhemispheric variant – syntelencephaly*
  - Non-separation of the posterior frontal and parietal regions
  - Normal anterior frontal and occipital lobes
  - Abnormal vertically oriented Sylvian fissure

Corpus Callosum Agenesis (CCA)

Corpus callosum is an interhemispheric association between the two cerebral hemispheres.

- Complete agenesis
- Partial agenesis (hypoplastic – anterior portion, including genu and anterior half of the body, is formed, but the posterior portion, including the posterior body and the rostrum, is not formed)
- Dysgenesis (malformed)

Risk factors: Maternal alcohol consumption during pregnancy, and maternal diabetes, along with male predilection.

CLINICAL

Dysmorphic facial features (hypertelorism and broad nose), hypotonia, learning disabilities, developmental delays, and seizures.

IMAGING

- Parallel orientation of ventricles on axial imaging
- Everted cingulate gyrus with small frontal horns (Viking helmet/moose-head appearance) in dysgenesis on a coronal scan

- Dilated, high-riding 3rd ventricle communicating with interhemispheric cistern, projecting as a dorsal cyst
- Colpocephaly (widened occipital horns of lateral ventricles – teardrop configuration)
- Absent septum pellucidum
- Absent cingulate gyrus and sulcus
- Lipomas

MANAGEMENT

Symptomatic, with psychomotor support, antiepileptics, psychotherapy.

Hemimegalencephaly

Unilateral hamartomatous enlargement of the cerebrum, which may, in some cases, cause ipsilateral cerebellar and brainstem enlargement (total hemimegalencephaly).

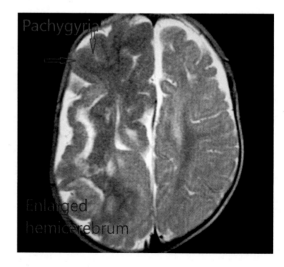

Figure 1.7 Hemimegalencephaly.

CLINICAL

Intractable seizures, hemiparesis contralateral to the affected hemisphere, and mental retardation.

IMAGING

CT and MRI:

- Enlarged hemicerebrum with focal polymicro-gyria, pachygyria, and lissencephaly to varying degrees
- Enlarged ipsilateral lateral ventricle with voluminous enlargement of the white matter (parenchyma)
- Thickened/dysplastic cortex, with an asymmetric enlargement of the vascular system, especially venous elements
- Indistinct gray–white matter interface
- Associated prominence of the cerebellar folia, and enlargement of the ipsilateral olfactory and optic nerve may be seen

DDs

- Hemimicrocephaly with asymmetric skull circumference
- Cerebral atrophy with symmetric skull circumference in Sturge-Weber syndrome
- Dyke-Davidoff-Masson syndrome
- Rasmussen encephalitis – chronic focal inflammatory disorder with unilateral cortical atrophy

MANAGEMENT

Antiepileptics, functional hemispherectomy.

ANCILLARY

Hemimegalencephaly has a syndromic association with the epidermal nevus syndrome, Proteus syndrome, hypomelanosis of Ito, Klippel-Trenaunay syndrome, and McCune-Albright syndrome.

Dyke-Davidoff-Masson Syndrome

Early brain insult results in hemicerebral atrophy.

CLINICAL

Seizures, contralateral hemiplegia.

IMAGING

- Cerebral hemiatrophy
- Ipsilateral compensatory skull vault thickening
- Hyperpneumatized frontal, ethmoid, and mastoid sinuses

DDs

Discussed under "Hemimegalencephaly."

Perisylvian Syndrome (Opercular Syndrome, Perisylvian Polymicrogyria, Worster-Drought Syndrome)

An organization/migration abnormality of the cortex of the perisylvian region, with multiple, anomalous, small convolutions and very few sulci – polymicrogyria. It usually occurs due to an *in utero* insult during the 5th or 6th month of pregnancy, and may be associated with congenital cytomegalovirus infection. The unilateral disease is a less severe form of its bilateral counterpart.

CLINICAL

Mental retardation, epilepsy and motor disturbances, oropharyngoglossal dysfunction, and dysarthria.

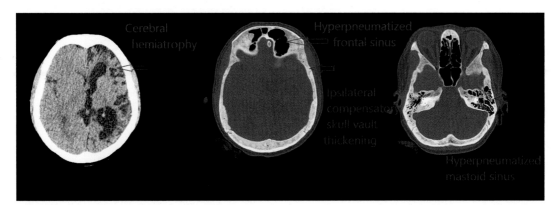

Figure 1.8 Dyke-Davidoff Masson syndrome.

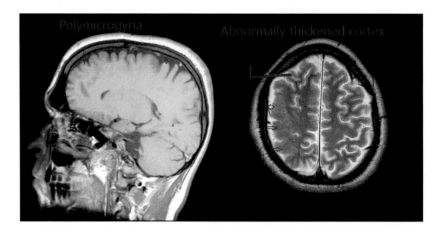

Figure 1.9 Right-sided perisylvian syndrome.

IMAGING

CT:

- Smooth thickening of the perisylvian cortex, with a cleft that may be seen in severe cases

MRI:

- Thickened cortex in the perisylvian region
- Poorly developed sulci with irregular margins at the cortical white matter junction
- Widened Sylvian fissure
- Inverted appearance of the bodies of the lateral ventricle

DDs

- Congenital Zika virus infection – bilateral and severe, with periventricular calcifications
- Pachygyria – thickened gyri with a reduced number of sulci

- Ulegyria, with characteristic mushroom-shaped gyri

MANAGEMENT

- Anticonvulsants, speech therapy, physical rehabilitation
- Surgical intervention (targeted focal corticectomy)

Hypoxic-Ischemic Encephalopathy (HIE/Hypoxic-Ischemic Injury)

HIE affects preterm (<36 weeks) or full-term (>36 weeks) neonates as a direct result of hypoxia, which, in turn, causes reduces blood flow to the brain (ischemia). Only hypoxemia without ischemia does not cause brain injury in neonates.

CLINICAL

Motor and cognitive developmental delays, seizures, paralysis and paraplegia, and cerebral palsy.

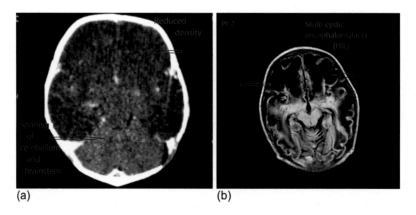

(a)   (b)

Figure 1.10 (a) White cerebellum sign, (b) multicystic encephalomalacia (HIE).

IMAGING

CT:

- Less-sensitive modality for evaluating HIE because of inadequate parenchymal contrast resolution due to the high water content of the brain parenchyma and the high protein content of the CSF in the neonatal brain, apart from the inherent drawback of radiation exposure
- *Reversal sign* – reversal in normal CT attenuation of gray matter and white matter
- *White cerebellum sign* – reduced density of cerebral cortical gray and white matter, loss of the gray–white matter interface, and the increased density of thalami, brainstem, and cerebellum suggest irreversible brain damage

MRI:

- Hypoxic-ischemic injury to gray matter – T1 hyperintensity and variable T2 intensity, depending on the time at imaging and the dominant underlying pathological condition, such as hemorrhage or gliosis
- Hypoxic-ischemic injury to white matter – T1 hypointensity and T2 hyperintensity due to ischemia-induced edema

DWI:

- Restricted diffusion in the perirolandic regions, corticospinal tracts, the ventrolateral thalamus, the globus pallidus, and putamen
- Corresponding ADC maps show a hypointensity that persists for a longer time than the hyperintensity of the DWI images

MR spectroscopy:

- Twin peak of high lactate levels, and low N-acetylaspartate (NAA) levels, with lactate: NAA ratio > 0.4

DDs

- Similar injury is seen in young children and adults as a result of choking, drowning, infections, or metabolic disorders
- Urea cycle defects – high peak serum glutamine
- Non-ketotic hyperglycemia in neonates presents with a high signal on DWI images, and a glycine peak on MRS

MANAGEMENT

Supportive and symptomatic management.

Porencephalic Cyst

Cystic, CSF-filled space that communicates with the ventricular system or the subarachnoid space (SAS) in the brain. They may be either congenital, due to ischemic insults or infection in the pre/perinatal period, or acquired (post-traumatic).

CLINICAL

Seizures, mental retardation, macrocephaly/microcephaly.

IMAGING

CT:

- Hypodense, non-enhancing cystic lesion

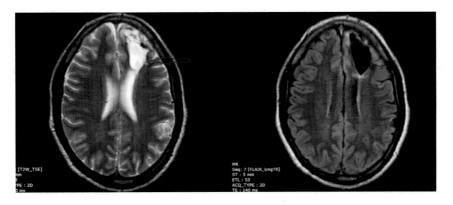

Figure 1.11 Porencephalic cyst.

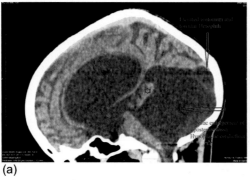
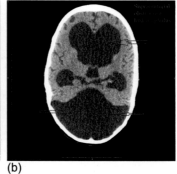

(a)   (b)

Figure 1.12 (a and b) Dandy-Walker malformation.

MRI:

- T2 hyperintense cystic lesion lined by white matter without any solid internal component

DDs

- Arachnoid cysts – extra-axial
- Neuroglial cysts – no communication with ventricles/SAS
- Schizencephaly – gray matter-lined cyst

MANAGEMENT

Anticonvulsants, speech therapy, and supportive measures.

ANCILLARY

Porencephalic cyst communicating with the ventricular system (internal cyst), with that communicating with the SAS (external cyst).

Dandy-Walker Malformation

Disorder involving the hindbrain.

CLINICAL

Macrocephaly, lack of motor coordination, and nystagmus.

IMAGING

Smooth, marginated, CSF-dense cystic lesion, with no contrast enhancement or calcification.

- Hypoplastic cerebellum and vermis
- Cystic enlargement of posterior fossa communicating with dilated 4th ventricle
- Supratentorial obstructive hydrocephalus

- Thinning and scalloping of the occipital bone
- Widely separated lambdoid sutures
- Displacement of tentorium and torcular Herophili above the lambdoid suture, with torcular lambdoid inversion
- Dysgenesis of corpus callosum and syringomyelia

DDs

- Dandy-Walker variant – vermian hypoplasia with cephalad rotation and possible 4th ventricle enlargement, but no posterior fossa enlargement
- Mega cisterna magna – enlarged cisterna magna (>10 mm) but normal cerebellum and vermis, with no hydrocephalus
- Persistent Blake's pouch cyst – cystic enlargement of the 4th ventricle through the foramen of Magendie, but with a normal cerebellum and vermis
- Retrocerebellar arachnoid cyst
- Cystic neoplasms – hemangioblastomas, pilocytic astrocytoma
- Joubert's syndrome

MANAGEMENT

Ventriculoperitoneal shunt, to reduce intracranial pressure.

Joubert's Syndrome

CLINICAL

Developmental delay, abnormal eye movements.

IMAGING

CT and MRI:

- Cerebellar vermis agenesis/hypoplastic

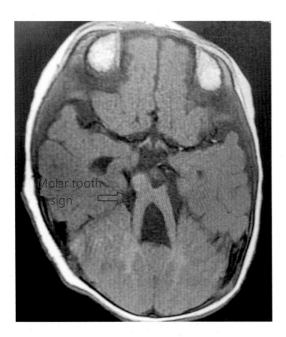

Figure 1.13 "Molar tooth" appearance.

- Molar tooth appearance of midbrain
  - Thickened, elongated, and dysplastic superior cerebellar peduncles
  - Deep interpeduncular fossa

- Bat-wing type 4th ventricle

DDs
- Dandy-Walker syndrome
- Rhombencephalosynapsis

MANAGEMENT
Genetic counseling.

SUGGESTED READING

Abdel Razek, AAK, Kandell, AY, Elsorogy, LG, Elmongy, A, Basett, AA. Disorders of cortical formation: MR imaging features. *AJNR Am J Neuroradiol* 2009;30(1):4–11.

Copeman, A, Jeanes, A, Young, J, Schelvan, C, Davis, J. *Paediatric Radiology for MRCPCH and FRCR.* 2nd ed. CRC Press; 2000.

Osborn, AG, Salzman, KL, Jhaveri, MD, Barkovich, AJ. *Diagnostic Imaging: Brain.* Elsevier Health Sciences; 2015.

Poe, LB, Coleman, LL, Mahmud, F. Congenital central nervous system anomalies. *Radiographics* 1989;9(5):801–826.

2

Vascular Anatomy

The bilateral internal carotid artery (ICA) and the vertebral artery (VA) supply blood to the brain. The Circle of Willis (CoW) is an interconnecting arterial polygon at the base of the brain, adjacent to the optic tract and the pituitary infundibulum. It consists of both anterior circulation (bilateral ICAs, the bilateral horizontal segment of the anterior communicating arteries [ACA] and the anterior communicating artery [AComA]) and posterior circulation (the basilar bifurcation, the bilateral horizontal segment of the posterior communicating arteries [PCA] and bilateral posterior communicating arteries [PComAs]).

INTERNAL CAROTID ARTERY – SEGMENTS AND THEIR BRANCHES

- C1 Cervical segment (extracranial branches
  - Carotid bulb
  - Cervical internal carotid artery
- C2 Petrous segment (intraosseous branches)
  - Tympanic branch
  - Vidian artery (artery of pterygoid canal)
  - Caroticotympanic branch
- C3 Lacerum segment
- C4 Cavernous segment
  - Meningohypophyseal artery
  - Inferolateral trunk
- C5 Supraclinoid segment
- C6 Ophthalmic segment
  - Ophthalmic artery
  - Superior hypophyseal artery
- C7 Communicating segment
  - Posterior communicating artery (PComA)
  - Anterior choroidal artery
  - Termination of ICA by bifurcation into the ACA and the middle cerebral artery (MCA)

Variants of ICA

CAROTID-VERTEBROBASILAR ANASTOMOSES

These are persistent embryonic circulatory channels between the caudal carotid artery and the vertebrobasilar arteries (embryonic paired longitudinal neural arteries), which fail to regress:

- The *persistent trigeminal artery* (PTA).
- The *persistent hypoglossal artery* (PHA) courses through the enlarged hypoglossal canal, parallels the 12th cranial nerve, and connects the cervical ICA with the basilar artery. It does not pass through the foramen magnum and may cause glossopharyngeal neuralgia.
- The *persistent dorsal ophthalmic artery* arises from the supraclinoid ICA, and traverses through the superior orbital fissure to the orbit instead of the optic canal.
- The *persistent primitive olfactory artery* normally regresses to the recurrent artery of Heubner. If it persists, it is associated with absent ACom artery and aneurysms.
- The *persistent otic artery* (POA).
- The *proatlantal intersegmental artery* (PIA) originates from the ICA/ECA and joins the vertebral artery at the C2–4 level, and passes through the foramen magnum.

PERSISTENT STAPEDIAL ARTERY (PSA)

The PSA originates from the petrous ICA, enclosed within the bony canal, and terminates as the middle meningeal artery. It may be associated with an enlarged facial nerve canal. CT scan shows the absence of the ipsilateral foramen spinosum. It may present with pulsatile tinnitus and needs to be differentiated from a glomus tympanicum tumor. It is pivotal to diagnose it preoperatively to avert such complications.

Aberrant ICA

Presents as a pulsatile retro/hypotympanic mass.

IMAGING

- Reduced diameter of ICA that courses posteriorly and parallel to the jugular bulb
- Bony dehiscence of the plate that separates the tympanic cavity from the ICA
- Vertical segment of the carotid canal
- Enlarged inferior tympanic canaliculus

DDs

- Glomus tympanicum paraganglioma
- Biopsy is contraindicated

Normal Variants

- Duplication is referred to as two discrete arteries with different origins and no confluence distally
- Fenestration is referred to as the division of the arterial lumen into two discrete channels,

which share the adventitia but have distinct endothelial and muscularis layers

CEREBRAL ARTERIES

Anterior Cerebral Artery (ACA)

- A1 (horizontal /pre-communicating segment) gives rise to medial lenticulostriate arteries
- A2 (distal/post-communicating segment)
  - Pericallosal
  - Callosomarginal
  - Recurrent artery of Heubner
  - Orbitofrontal
  - Frontopolar
- A3 – cortical branches supply the anterior two-thirds of the medial hemispheric surface and a small superior area extending over the convexities
- Anterior communicating artery (AComA) completes the COW anteriorly by joining two ACAs

VARIANTS AND ANOMALIES

- Hypoplastic/absent A1 segment of ACA
- Duplicated or absent AComA

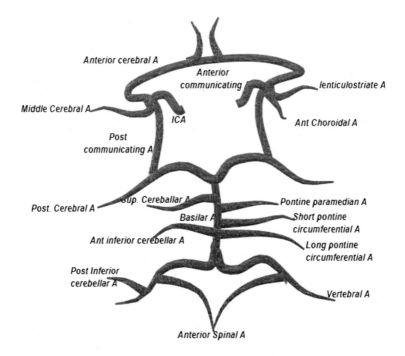

Figure 2.1 Circle of Willis.

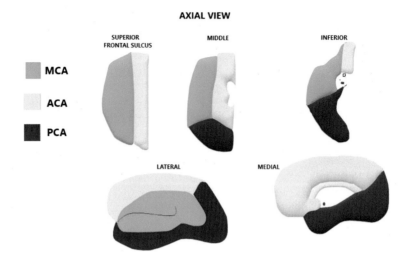

Figure 2.2 Territorial distribution of major arteries.

- Trifurcation of ACA due to the persistence of the median callosal artery
- Azygous ACA – a solitary unpaired vessel that arises due to the persistence of the embryonic median artery of the corpus callosum and supplies the bilateral anterior cerebral hemispheres. It may be associated with intracranial aneurysms, holoprosencephaly, and other neuronal migration anomalies

Middle Cerebral Artery (MCA)

- M1 (horizontal segment) – gives rise to lateral lenticulostriate arteries that supply most of the basal ganglia
- M2 – insular segment
- M3 – opercular/Sylvian segment
- M4 – cortical segment

VARIANTS

- Accessory MCA arising from ACA and simulating duplicated MCA.

Posterior Cerebral Artery (PCA)

- P1 – Pre-communicating segment (peduncular branches)
  - Posterior thalamoperforating arteries
  - Medial posterior choroidal artery
- P2 – Ambient (post-communicating) segment
  - Lateral posterior choroidal arteries
  - Thalamogeniculate arteries

- P3 – Quadrigeminal segment
  - Inferior temporal artery
  - Parieto-occipital artery
  - Calcarine artery
  - Posterior pericallosal (splenial) artery

VARIANTS

- Hypoplasia of one or both PComA.
- Fetal origin of PCA from ICA with hypoplastic/absent P1 PCA.
- Infundibular dilatation at the PComA – funnel-shaped/conical dilatation at the origin of the PComA from the ICA. An infundibulum must be differentiated from aneurysms of the PComA and ICA.
- Common origin of the posterior cerebral and superior cerebellar arteries.

VERTEBROBASILAR SYSTEM

VAs are usually 3–5 mm in diameter and arise from the subclavian arteries bilaterally. They divide into the following segments:

- V1 from the origin to the transverse foramen of the sixth cervical vertebra
- V2 from the transverse foramen of the sixth cervical vertebra to that of the second cervical vertebra
- V3 from the transverse foramen of the second cervical vertebra to the dura
- V4 from the dura to the basilar artery

Right and left VAs unite to form the basilar artery (BA, 3 cm in length and up to 4 mm in width, normally) near the pontomedullary junction.

Vertebral Artery

- Anterior spinal artery
- Posterior inferior cerebellar artery (PICA)

Basilar Artery

- Anterior inferior cerebellar artery (AICA)
- Superior cerebellar artery (SCA)
- Perforating branches
- Terminates into two posterior cerebral arteries (PCAs) in interpeduncular fossa

VARIANTS

- Hypoplastic/duplicated/fenestrated VAs
- Origin of left VA from aortic arch
- Non-fused BA
- Persistent vertebrobasilar anastomosis
- Anomalous origin of PICA from extracranial VA below the foramen magnum

Venous Anatomy

- Dural sinuses
- Superficial cortical veins
- Deep cerebral veins

Cerebral veins are valveless, thin-walled, and have no muscular tissue.

Dural Sinuses

These are the venous channels located between the endosteal and meningeal layers of the dura mater.

UNPAIRED SINUSES

- The superior sagittal sinus (SSS) is the largest dural venous sinus, and lies in the midline between the inner table of the skull (superiorly) and the falx cerebri (laterally)
- The inferior sagittal sinus lies in the inferior free margin of the falx cerebri
- The straight sinus (SS)
- The occipital sinus, the smallest dural venous sinus, is important to identify during posterior fossa craniotomy
- The inter-cavernous sinus

PAIRED SINUSES

- The transverse sinus (TS).
- Sigmoid sinuses – inferior continuation of the TS, which continue inferiorly into the jugular bulb at the skull base.
- The superior petrosal sinus (SPS).
- The inferior petrosal sinus (IPS).
- The sphenoparietal sinus.

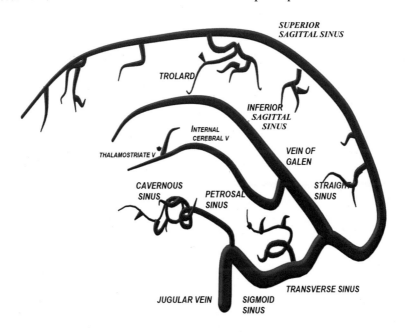

Figure 2.3 Venous anatomy.

- Cavernous sinuses – complex, multi-septate venous spaces lateral to the sella. They receive the superior ophthalmic vein (SOV) and the inferior ophthalmic vein (IOV) and communicate with each other *via* an inter-cavernous sinus.

Torcula Herophili – confluence of sinuses overlying the internal occipital protuberance.

Superficial Cortical Veins

Most are not named but are known as superior, middle, and inferior cerebral veins. Only three can be identified:

- Superficial middle cerebral vein that runs along the Sylvian fissure
- Vein of Trolard, the largest cortical vein, drains into the SSS
- Vein of Labbe, which drains the temporal lobe

Deep Cerebral Veins

Easily identified on late venous phase cerebral angiograms:

- Medullary veins drain subcortical and deep white matter. These usually get enlarged in vascular malformations, collateral channels, vascular neoplasms, etc.
- Subependymal veins surround the lateral ventricles and receive blood from medullary veins.
- The thalamostriate vein and septal vein join to form internal cerebral veins (ICVs), which are paired median structures that lie just above the roof of the 3rd ventricle in the velum interpositum.
- Basal veins of Rosenthal (BVoR) run in the ambient cistern posterosuperiorly.
- Great cerebral vein of Galen (VOG) curves posteriorly under the splenium of corpus callosum. The ICVs and BVoR drain into the VOG. With the inferior sagittal sinus, it joins the straight sinus, which then drains into the torcula Herophili.

VARIANTS AND PITFALLS

- Hypoplastic/asymmetric transverse sinus.
- Atresia of one-third of the superior sagittal sinus.

- A flow gap, if seen in the transverse sinus and the transverse-sigmoid junction, should not be mistaken for a thrombus.
- Arachnoid granulations and partial split SSS may mimic a thrombus.
- Persistent falcine sinus refers to the recanalization of the fetal falcine sinus due to the absence or thrombosis of the SSS. Normally, the falcine sinus is seen in falx cerebri of the fetus and involutes after birth.

Stroke

Since the brain is sensitive to hypoxia, neurological deficits may occur due to disturbance in the blood supply to the brain, causing a cerebrovascular accident (CVA). It progresses sequentially from ischemia (reduced blood flow) to frank infarction (complete vessel occlusion).

ETIOLOGY

- Thrombosis due to a clot in the blood vessel
- Embolism due to an obstruction of the blood vessels by an embolism elsewhere in the body
- Hemorrhage due to blood accumulation in the cranial cavity
- Hypoperfusion due to lack of blood supply to the brain

Major types of stroke:

- Infarction
- Intracerebral hemorrhage
- Subarachnoid hemorrhage
- Venous occlusions

IMAGING

Angiography

- Occluded vessel
- Slow antegrade filling, with delayed arterial emptying
- Collaterals
- Vascular blush due to luxury perfusion

MRI

- Reduced N-acetylaspartate (NAA) and elevated lactate levels
- Typical "rapid stroke" sequence includes a FLAIR, DWI, ADC, and GRE, which help to detect foci of blood, usually seen as a susceptibility artifact

Table 2.1 Imaging Features of Stroke during Different Phases

	Hyperacute (< 12 hours)	Acute (12–24 hours)	Early Subacute (< 1 week)	Late Subacute (1–8 weeks)	Chronic (months–years)
NCCT	May be normal Hyperdense artery Obscuration of lentiform nuclei	Loss of GWM interface Effaced sulci Hypodense basal ganglia	Mass effect Edema Wedge-shaped hypodensity involving both GM and WM Hemorrhagic transformation (HT) may occur	Mass effect subsides	Volume loss with encephalomalacia (hypodense areas) and *ex vacuo* ventriculomegaly
CECT			Gyral enhancement	Enhancement may be seen	
MRI	Absent normal flow void T1WI better delineates: Effaced sulci Gyral edema Loss of GWM interface	T2 hyperintense signal of the affected region	Reducing mass effect and edema HT may occur	Mass effect subsides	Volume loss with encephalomalacia Wallerian degeneration with ipsilateral brainstem atrophy
CE-MRI	Intravascular contrast enhancement	Meningeal enhancement adjacent to the afflicted region	Parenchymal contrast enhancement Intravascular and meningeal enhancement subsides	Parenchymal contrast enhancement	
DWI	High (restriction seen)	High	Gradual decrease	Gradual decrease	Low
ADC	Low	Low	Gradual increase	Gradual increase	High

Stroke in Children

ETIOLOGY

- Cerebral emboli from congenital heart disease with right to left shunts
- Traumatic or spontaneous dissection of the internal carotid or vertebral arteries
- Moyamoya disease (idiopathic progressive arteriopathy)
- Infection (tonsillitis, meningitis)
- Hypoxia
- Sickle cell disease
- Neurofibromatosis 1
- Drug abuse (amphetamines, cocaine, etc.)

Stroke Mimics

- MELAS (Mitochondrial myopathy, Encephalopathy, Lactic Acidosis, Stroke-like episodes). Differentiating features include non-vascular distribution, multifocal lesions, and propensity to involve posterior parietal and occipital lobes.
- Hemiplegic migraine may also show restricted diffusion, but can be differentiated by non-vascular distribution, no vascular occlusion, and long histories of migraine.
- Metabolic hypoglycemia may produce a stroke-like picture, with hemiplegia and aphasia.

Bedside laboratory testing for glucose should be expedited for diagnosis. Administration of intravenous glucose may treat the hemiplegia, which may resolve.

- Herpes simplex encephalitis
- Seizures and postictal status (Todd's paresis). Transient nature of clinical and imaging features.
- Tumors.

INTRACRANIAL ANEURYSMS

Focal dilatation/outpouchings of intracranial vessels occur, usually at arterial bifurcation points. They can be multiple and occur at a higher frequency in females. They can be saccular, fusiform, or dissecting. True aneurysms refer to the dilatation of the vessel lumen, owing to the weakness of all four layers of the vessel wall.

Etiology

- Developmental/degenerative
- Atherosclerotic
- Underlying vasculopathy-like arteritis, fibromuscular dysplasia, dissection
- Flow related within the nidus of arterial-venous malformations (AVMs)
- Traumatic
- Infection (mycotic)
- Neoplasm (oncotic)

- Critical size for aneurysm rupture is between 4 and 7 mm
- Giant aneurysm >2.5 cm may produce symptoms due to mass effect

INTRACRANIAL VASCULAR MALFORMATIONS

1) Pial (parenchymal), dural, or mixed AVM
2) Venous malformations (DVA/venous angioma, VOGM, varix)
3) Cavernous angioma
4) Capillary telangiectasia

CASE STUDIES

ICA Aneurysm

CLINICAL

Asymptomatic/nerve palsies, seizures, headaches, temporary ischemic attacks (TIAs). Subarachnoid hemorrhage (SAH) is the most frequent presentation. It may result in vasospasm, leading to deficits and death.

IMAGING

See Table 2.3.

MANAGEMENT

Endovascular repair.

Table 2.2 Features Differentiating between Stroke and Tumor

Stroke	Tumor
Sudden onset	Gradual onset
Wedge shaped	Round/lobulated or infiltrating
Involves both gray and white matter	Affects the white matter and tends to spare the cortex
Typical vascular territory	Non-vascular distribution

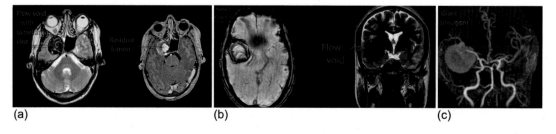

(a) (b) (c)

Figure 2.4 (a) Partially thrombosed aneurysm, (b and c) giant ICA aneurysm.

Table 2.3 Imaging Findings of Patent and Thrombosed Aneurysms

	Patent Aneurysm	Partially Thrombosed Aneurysm	Completely Thrombosed Aneurysm
NCCT	Well defined iso- to hyperdense lesion located eccentrically in the subarachnoid space/fissures	Patent lumen inside the thick/multilamellar/calcified wall	Hyperdense
CECT	Intense homogeneous enhancement	Residual lumen and outer rim may enhance	No increased attenuation
MRI (aneurysm with rapid flow)	Flow void (signal loss on both T1 and T2W) Only wall enhancement may be seen	Flow void surrounded by concentric layers of lamellated clot	Subacute thrombus is hyperintense on T1 and T2WI Multilayered clots with variable intensity due to repeated hemorrhages of varying ages
MRI (aneurysm with slow/turbulent flow)	Signal heterogeneity and variable enhancement may be seen	Residual lumen is isointense	

Ruptured ACom Aneurysm

CLINICAL

Worst headache ever, unconsciousness.

IMAGING

SAH-CT hyperdensity and FLAIR hyperintensity that spread within cisterns/subarachnoid spaces in the acute stage.

Aneurysmal irregularity and vasospasm.

MANAGEMENT

Endovascular repair.

Post-coiling imaging. Hypointensity at the site of the previously known aneurysm on MR angiography.

ANCILLARY

- Blood in Sylvian fissure suggests ipsilateral ICA, PComA, MCA aneurysm
- Focal interhemispheric blood suggests AComA aneurysm

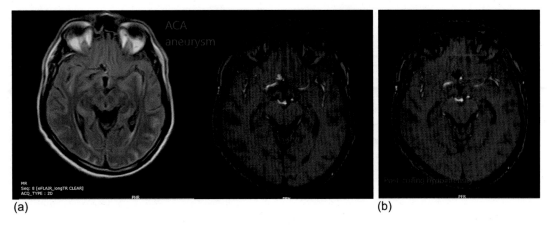

Figure 2.5 (a) Ruptured ACom aneurysm, (b) post-coiling hypointensity.

- 4th ventricle hemorrhage suggests PICA aneurysm

Basilar Tip Aneurysm

Basilar tip aneuryms occur at the distal bifurcation of the basilar artery, between the origin of the two posterior cerebral arteries.

CLINICAL

SAH, compressive neuropathies, altered state of consciousness. Progressive headache may precede the rupture of a saccular aneurysm.

IMAGING

- NCCT – SAH, curvilinear calcification, and thrombosis
- CECT – surrounding edema and inflammatory reaction
- CTA – morphology of aneurysm, its diameter, and its relationship to the parent vessel
- MRI – aneurysmal flow voids, adjacent heterogeneous signal intensity due to thrombi of varying ages
- FLAIR – SAH

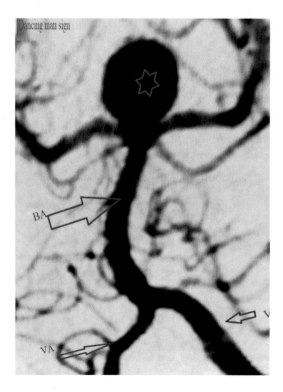

Figure 2.6 Basilar tip aneurysm.

- Phase contrast (PC) MRA – detection of flow patterns and slow flow, especially in giant aneurysms
- Time-of-flight (TOF) – for small aneurysms
- Conventional angiography – gold standard for the detection and evaluation of the location, size, and morphology of basilar tip aneurysms ("dancing man" sign)
- Digital subtraction angiography with bi-planar magnification views
  - Aneurysmal irregularity, daughter loculus, or focal spasm (suggests acute rupture)
  - Vasospasm and the collateral circulation

MANAGEMENT

Surgery – for symptomatic/ruptured aneurysms with surgical clips/coils (endovascular techniques).
    Supportive treatment for candidates unsuited for surgery.

Cavernoma

These are discrete, lobulated, multiple hamartomatous lesions formed by sinusoidal vascular spaces, without intervening cerebral parenchyma, and containing hemorrhages in different stages of evolution. They are most often supratentorial, located in the deep cortical white matter, basal ganglia, and at the corticomedullary junction. Pons and cerebellar hemispheres are the most common infratentorial locations.

CLINICAL

Seizures, neurologic defects, headaches.

IMAGING

- NCCT– isodense to hyperdense foci, often with calcifications and no mass effect or edema.
- CECT – minimal enhancement.
- Angiographically occult.
- MRI – classic "popcorn" lesion with a complex core of mixed-signal intensities, representing various stages of evolving hemorrhage.
  - Low-signal hemosiderin ring completely surrounds the angioma, which becomes more prominent (darker) on T2 and gradient-echo images. Because of this "blooming effect," GRE should be performed when a solitary hemorrhagic lesion is identified

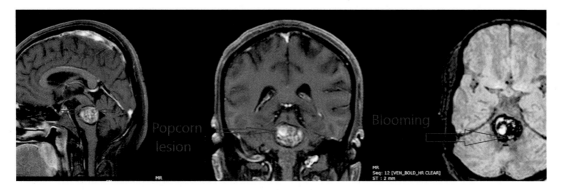

Figure 2.7 Pontine cavernoma and blooming effect.

to exclude the presence of multiple lesions (which may not be visible on standard spin-echo sequences).

DDs

- Tumors – usually, do not have complete hemosiderin rings
- Simple hemorrhage – often, collapse into slit-like cavities, but cavernomas maintain their rounded shape

MANAGEMENT

- Antiepileptics
- Surgical resection

ANCILLARY

Venous angiomas occur most frequently in conjunction with cavernous angiomas

Developmental Venous Anomaly (DVA)/Venous Angioma

Dysplastic superficial or deep cerebral veins result in dilatation of transmedullary veins, which converge into large draining veins and then into deep venous systems. Intervening brain parenchyma is normal.

CLINICAL

Asymptomatic.

IMAGING

- NCCT – normal/slightly hyperdense ill-defined area, due to thrombosis of draining vein, simulating subarachnoid hemorrhage
  - No edema and mass effect
- CECT – tuft of enhancing vessels near ventricle
  - Dilated draining vein

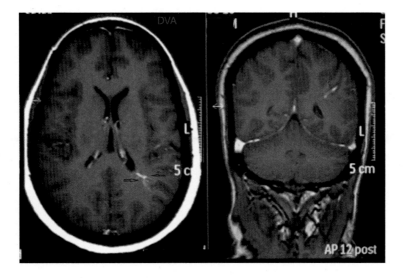

Figure 2.8 Developmental venous anomaly.

- MRI – flow voids on T1 and T2
  - T1 hyperintensity (clot in the draining vein)
- FLAIR – adjacent hyperintensity due to edema and infarction
- CE-MRI – intensely enhancing a stellate tangle of medullary tributaries
  - Dilated subependymal draining vein
- Angiography – arterial phase: normal
  - Capillary phase: blush
  - Venous phase: Medusa head of enlarged medullary veins and enlarged transcortical or subependymal draining veins

COMPLICATION

Thrombosed DVA → venous hypertension → venous infarct and intracranial hemorrhage

Arteriovenous Malformations (AVMs)

This involves direct communication of arteries to veins without an intervening capillary bed and is a frequent cause of unexplained intracranial hemorrhage in a child or normotensive young adult.

CLINICAL

Seizures, headache, neurological deficits.

IMAGING

See Table 2.4.

MANAGEMENT

Endovascular, surgical, or radiation.

Vein of Galen Malformation

Developmental malformation with an A-V shunt in the wall of an embryologic venous precursor median vein of the prosencephalon (MVP) of Markowski and its aneurysmal dilatation. The dilated MVP drains *via* the dural sinuses.

CLINICAL

High-output cardiac failure, macrocephaly.

IMAGING

- NCCT – mildly hyperdense lesion in the midline within the cistern of the velum interpositum
- CECT – enhances intensely
- MRI – large flow void in the midline on T1 and T2WI
- DWI – restricted diffusion in regions of associated infarction
- CT/MR angiography/venography – feeding arteries and the varix drainage for embolization planning

DDs

- Intracranial vascular tumor
- Intracranial AVM

MANAGEMENT

Endovascular staged embolization.

ANCILLARY

VOGM refers to an arteriovenous fistula between the deep choroidal arteries and the embryonic median prosencephalic vein of Markowski. It is associated with persistent falcine sinus and can be

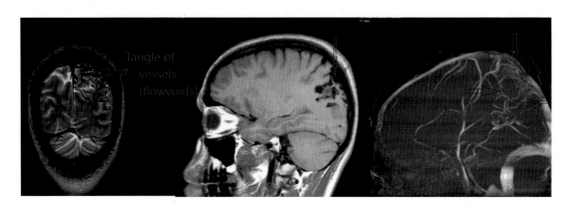

Figure 2.9 Tangle of vessels (flow voids).

Table 2.4 Imaging Findings of Patent and Thrombosed Brain AVMs and Dural Malformations

	NCCT	CECT	MRI	Angiography
Patent brain AVMs	Iso- to hyperdense serpiginous vessels	Intense enhancement	Tightly packed flow voids (high-velocity signal loss) T2 hyperintense signal due to gliosis Blood products of various stages	Enlarged feeding arteries and veins AV shunting Early draining veins Nidus
Thrombosed brain AVMs	Calcification may be noted	Variable enhancement	Heterogeneous signal intensity	Stagnant flow Subtle AV shunting
Dural AVM/Fs	Usually normal Enlarged dural sinus Venous varix	Dilated superior ophthalmic vein in carotico-cavernous fistula	Dilated cortical veins without any identifiable nidus PC-MRA can delineate flow direction in draining veins and dural sinuses	Enlarged dural arteries AV shunting Dural sinus stenosis

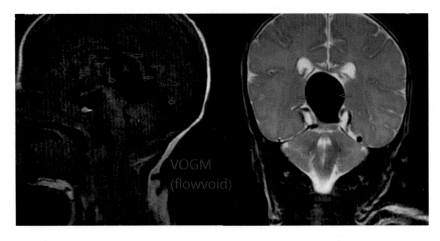

Figure 2.10 Vein of Galen malformation.

categorized into choroidal and mural subtypes (see Table 2.5).

Cirsoid Aneurysm of Scalp (Plexiform Angioma)

Arteriovenous malformations (fistula); can be congenital or post-traumatic.

CLINICAL

Slow-growing pulsatile mass, bruit, headache.

IMAGING
- NCCT – serpiginous subcutaneous lesion
- CECT – marked enhancement of tangle of vessels
- Angiography – feeders from superficial temporal, occipital, or supraorbital arteries, and drainage through scalp veins

DDs
- Soft tissue venous malformation (hemangioma)
- Metastasis from follicular carcinoma thyroid
- Pseudoaneurysm
- Sinus pericranii

MANAGEMENT

Endovascular occlusion
  Surgical resection

Anterior Cerebral Artery Infarct

Less common, because of collateral flow through the contralateral side if the A1 segment of one side develops thrombosis.

CLINICAL

Contralateral motor weakness of the leg, contralateral cortical sensory deficit, dysarthria, impaired judgment, urinary incontinence, aphasia.

IMAGING

ACA stroke mainly involves the frontoparietal cerebral cortex (paramedian), the corpus callosum (anteriorly), the caudate head (inferiorly), and the internal capsule (anterior limb).

Table 2.5 Features Differentiating between Choroidal and Mural Type VOGM

Choroidal Type	Mural Type
Neonates	Infants and children
High-output cardiac failure	Developmental delay and hydrocephalus
Supplied by multiple feeding vessels from the pericallosal, choroidal, and thalamoperforating arteries	Supplied by a single or a few feeders from the collicular or posterior choroidal arteries

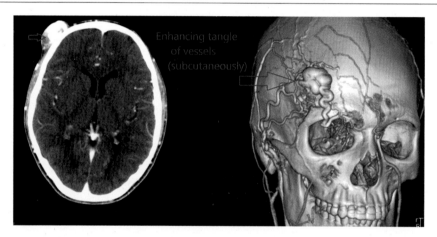

Figure 2.11 Cirsoid aneurysm.

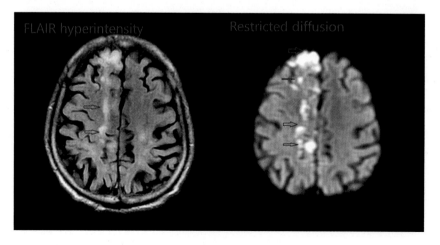

Figure 2.12 ACA territory infarct.

- NCCT – hypodensity involving gray and white matter, with loss of gray–white matter differentiation. Detects hemorrhage, if any
- MRI – hypointense on T1WI and hyperintense on T2WI
- DWI – restricts and identifies ischemia within thirty minutes of onset; much earlier than CT
- GRE – thrombus and microbleed blooming
- MR perfusion – DWI-PWI and CBV-CBF mismatch to estimate penumbra
- Angiography – delineates thrombus and area of non-perfused brain

DDs

See "Stroke Mimics."

MANAGEMENT

- Intra-arterial or intravenous thrombolysis
- Mechanical thrombectomy

Middle Cerebral Artery (MCA) Infarct

MCA supplies a portion of the frontal, temporal, and parietal lobes, controlling primary motor and sensory areas of the face, throat, hand, and arm, and speech.

CLINICAL

Contralateral hemiparesis, hemisensory loss, hemianopia, and aphasia.

IMAGING

- NCCT – insular ribbon sign
  - Hyperdense vessel sign
  - Mass effect with sulcal effacement
- CT angiography – abrupt occlusion of the vessel with enhancement of distal vasculature absent
- MRI – low signal on T1W and high signal on T2W and FLAIR, along with restricted diffusion on DWI
- DWI-PWI and CBV-CBF mismatch on MR perfusion images
- DSA aids in the identification of a thrombus and the area of non-perfused brain

Chronic infarct – hypodense areas of encephalomalacia/gliosis with mild *ex vacuo* dilatation of lateral ventricle.

DDs

See "Stroke Mimics."

MANAGEMENT

- Intravenous or intra-arterial thrombolysis
- Endovascular thrombectomy

Posterior Cerebral Artery Infarct

CLINICAL

Contralateral homonymous hemianopia (due to occipital lobe infarction), hemisensory loss, and hemi-body pain (due to thalamic infarction).

IMAGING

See Table 2.1.

- NCCT – hypodensity involving gray and white matter in the occipital lobe, with loss of gray–white matter differentiation
- CT angiography – abrupt occlusion of the vessel with enhancement of distal vasculature absent
- MRI – low signal on T1W and high signal on T2W and FLAIR, along with restricted diffusion on DWI

DWI-PWI and CBV-CBF mismatch on MR perfusion images help in estimating penumbra.

DSA aids in identification of thrombus and area of non-perfused brain.

DDs

See "Stroke Mimics."

MANAGEMENT

Thrombolysis/thrombectomy.

Artery of Percheron Infarct

The artery of Percheron is an anatomical variant of the posterior circulation in which a single common trunk arises from the first segment of either the left or right posterior cerebral artery (P1), that supplies the thalamus and midbrain bilaterally. Risk factors include hypertension, diabetes, and atrial fibrillation, which result in infarction secondary to occlusion of the artery of Percheron, due to atherosclerosis or embolism.

CLINICAL

Altered mental status, vertical gaze palsy, memory impairment, hypersomnolence, hemiplegia, sensory disturbances, and cognitive impairments.

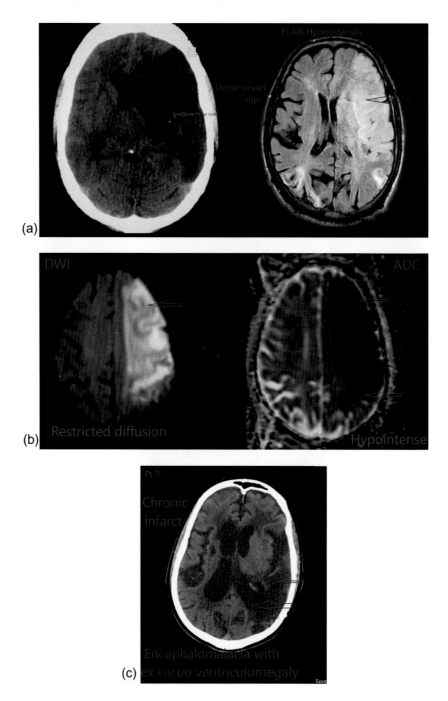

Figure 2.13 (a and b) Large left-sided MCA territory infarct, (c) chronic infarct.

IMAGING

- CT – hypodensities of bilateral paramedian thalamus and rostral midbrain
- MRI –T1 hypointense and T2/FLAIR hyperintense signal with some patchy heterogeneous enhancement
- T2/FLAIR – V-shaped hyperintense signal along the pial surface of the midbrain at the posterior wall of the interpeduncular fossa ("midbrain V sign")
- DWI – restricted diffusion is noted

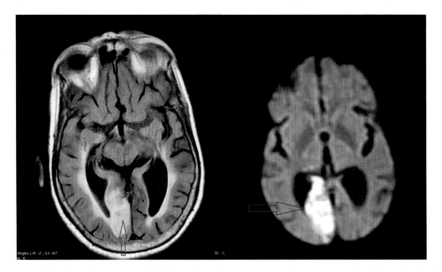

Figure 2.14 (a and b) Right-sided PCA infarct.

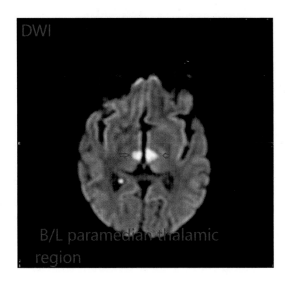

DWI

B/L paramedian thalamic region

Figure 2.15 Artery of Percheron infarct.

DDs

- Top of the basilar artery syndrome – infarction of the thalamus, along with occlusion of posterior circulation, affect the midbrain and portions of the temporal and occipital lobes
- Deep cerebral venous thrombosis – ischemia in the thalamus, but it will also involve the internal capsule and basal ganglia
- Other diagnoses that cause thalamic restriction of DWI include Wernicke's encephalopathy, Creutzfeldt-Jakob disease, metabolic or toxic processes, and bilateral thalamic glioma

MANAGEMENT

- Thrombolysis
- Intravenous heparin, long-term anticoagulant usage, and rehabilitation

Posterior Inferior Cerebellar Artery (PICA) Infarct – Lateral Medullary Syndrome (Wallenberg Syndrome)

The territory of PICA includes the lateral medulla, the inferior cerebellum, and the vermis.

CLINICAL

Nausea, vomiting, ataxia, and vertigo (involvement of the vestibular system).

IMAGING

- CT – less sensitive due to artifacts caused by the bony structures surrounding the brainstem and cerebellum
- CT angiography helps in delineating occluded and dolichoectatic vessels
- MRI – low signal on T1W and high signal on T2W and FLAIR, along with restricted diffusion on DWI

MANAGEMENT

Thrombolysis.

Watershed (Border Zone) Infarct

Located between major vascular territories.

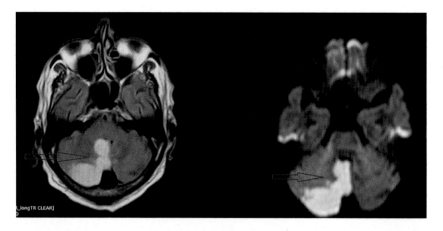

Figure 2.16 Right-sided PICA infarct.

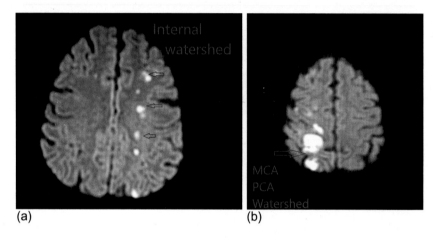

(a)   (b)

Figure 2.17 (a) Internal watershed infarcts, (b) external watershed infarct.

CLINICAL

Hemiparesis, seizures.

IMAGING

- CT – appear hypodense on CT
- MRI – hypointense on T1WI, hyperintense on T2W/ FLAIR, and show restricted diffusion on DWI (see Table 2.6)

Lacunar Infarct

Small infarcts (<1.5–2.0 cm) in the deeper parts of the basal ganglia, internal capsule, thalamus, white matter, and brainstem, caused by stenosis of the deep penetrating artery.

CAUSES

- Hypertension
- Atherosclerosis
- Emboli

CLINICAL

TIA, hemiparesis.

IMAGING

- CT – appears hypodense on CT
- MRI – follows CSF signal intensity
- DWI – shows restricted diffusion

DDs

- Dilated Virchow-Robin spaces
- Neurocysticercosis

Cerebral Venous Thrombosis

Pivotal cause of stroke in children and young adults. The risk factors include dehydration, trauma pregnancy, a hypercoagulable state, and adjacent infection (e.g., mastoiditis).

Table 2.6 Differentiation between External and Internal Watershed Infarcts

External/Cortical	Internal/Deep White Matter
Emboli, hypoperfusion	Hemodynamic compromise, severe stenosis
Between ACA, MCA, and PCA territories	Between ACA, MCA, and PCA territories and perforating lenticulostriate, thalamoperforating, anterior choroidal arteries, etc.
Wedge-shaped/gyriform in frontal cortex (ACA-MCA) and parieto-occipital region (MCA-PCA)	Confluent or band-like linear lesions in the centrum semiovale or corona radiata, parallel to ventricles
Marked hypoperfusion–parallel parafalcine stripes in the subcortical white matter at the vertex	
Less morbidity	High morbidity

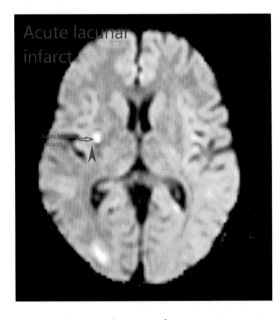

Figure 2.18 Acute lacunar infarct.

CLINICAL

Headache, seizures, unconsciousness.

IMAGING

- NCCT – hyperdense dural venous sinus (dense clot sign) or cortical veins (cord sign)
- MRI – loss of flow void (iso- to hyperintense) on T1 and T2WI
- CECT – empty delta sign, enhancing dural collateral circulation, surrounding the non-enhancing thrombosed sinus (especially the superior sagittal sinus)
- CT/MR venogram – filling defect within the sinus
- GRE – blooming (susceptibility hypointensity) within the thrombosed venous sinus/cortical vein
- Angiography – non-filling of veins

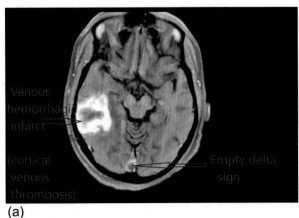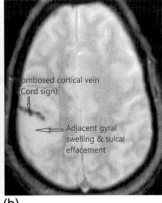

(a) (b)

Figure 2.19 (a) Empty delta sign with venous infarct, (b) cord sign.

PITFALLS

- Arachnoid granulations
- Slow flow
- Hypoplastic sinus (normal variant)

MANAGEMENT

Catheter-directed thrombolysis.

Venous Infarct with Dural Sinus Thrombosis

CLINICAL

Headache, seizures.

IMAGING

- CT – hypodensity, T1 hypointensity, T2/FLAIR hyperintensity in the subcortical white matter, usually paramedian location, not following any arterial territory. Associated linear hyperdensities on CT suggest hemorrhagic nature of the infarct.
- CECT/ MRI – enhancement +/–
- DWI – usually not seen (T2 shine-through may be seen)

- Sinus thrombosis as described in the previous case

DDs

- Low-grade gliomas
- Encephalitis

MANAGEMENT

Anticoagulation/ thrombectomy.

Moyamoya Disease

Rare cerebrovascular occlusive disease-causing bilateral occlusion of the supraclinoid portion of the ICA, that extends to the proximal portions of the ACA and the MCA. It is associated with parenchymal, leptomeningeal, or transdural collateral vessels that supply the ischemic brain. It is more common in the Japanese population and in children.

CLINICAL

- Children – headaches, seizures, behavioral disturbances, and recurrent hemiparetic attacks
- Adults – bleeding or strokes

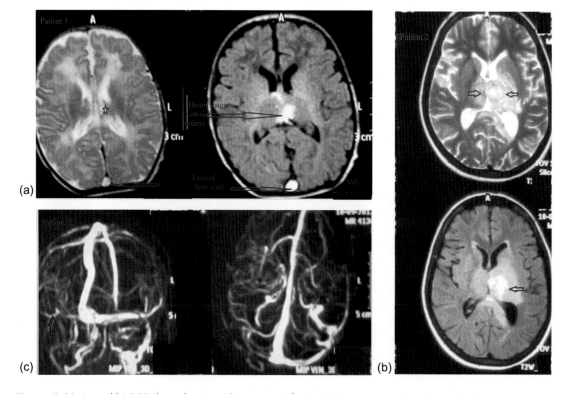

Figure 2.20 (a and b) SSS thrombosis with venous infarct, (c) transverse sinus thrombosis.

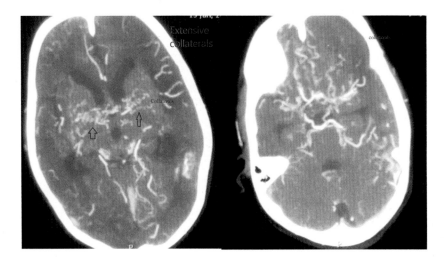

Figure 2.21 Moyamoya disease.

IMAGING

- Angiography/CTA/MRA
- Stenosis or occlusion of supraclinoid ICA
- "Puff of smoke" appearance, with numerous collaterals supplying the ACA and MCA distribution, which often anastomoses between the leptomeningeal and dural meningeal arteries
- MRI – chronic ischemic changes, including atrophy, gliosis, and prominent ventricles

MANAGEMENT

Surgical treatment – encephaloduroarteriosynangiosis (EDAS).

Cerebral Autosomal Dominant Arteriopathy with Subcortical Infarcts and Leukoencephalopathy (CADASIL)

Genetic microvasculopathy characterized by lacunar and subcortical white matter strokes and vascular dementia in younger patients, owing to arteriopathy affecting penetrating cerebral and leptomeningeal arteries. It classically involves the anterior temporal pole, the paramedian frontal lobe, and the external capsule with relative sparing of cortical gray matter, subcortical U-fibers, and the occipital and orbitofrontal regions.

CLINICAL

Recurrent TIA/stroke (most common), cognitive decline, migraine.

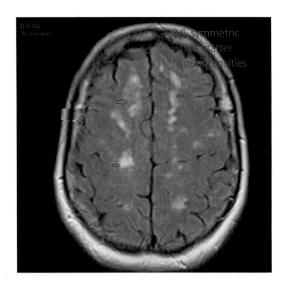

Figure 2.22 Bilateral WMHs of CADASIL.

IMAGING

- CT – hypodensities at a characteristic location
- MRI-T2/FLAIR – non-enhancing, multifocal, bilateral, symmetric white matter hyperintensities (WMHs) throughout subcortical, periventricular, and deep white matter, as well as lacunar infarcts in deep gray structures. Cerebral atrophy in later stages
- DWI – diffusion restriction in acute/subacute infarcts
- GRE and SWI – cerebral microhemorrhages
- Normal cerebral angiogram

DDs

- Multi-infarct/vascular dementia
- Multiple sclerosis – contrast enhancement of the active lesions, the involvement of optic nerve and spinal cord, and no microbleeds
- Atherosclerotic stroke
- Susac syndrome involves corpus callosum mainly
- MELAS

MANAGEMENT

Symptomatic therapy with psychological and physical rehabilitation, antiplatelet drugs, statins.

ANCILLARY

Consider CADASIL in a young patient with cerebral white matter disease, especially when there is no history of vascular disease, radiation/chemotherapy, demyelinating disease, or an immunocompromised state.

Posterior Reversible Encephalopathy Syndrome (PRES)

Usually seen in patients with preeclampsia/eclampsia, post solid organ transplant, sepsis.

CLINICAL

Moderate to severe hypertension, visual changes, nausea, altered mental status, and paresis.

IMAGING

- CT – bilateral, hypodense areas involving posterior circulation.

- MRI – bilateral, patchy cortical/subcortical hyperintensity (vasogenic edema) on T2/FLAIR, mainly involving posterior parietal/occipital lobes, cortical watershed zones, and cerebellum with variable contrast enhancement. No restricted diffusion on DWI.
- Angiography may show signs of vasospasm or arteritis with multifocal segmental arterial constriction, giving "string of beads" appearance.

DDs

- Acute ischemia/infarct exhibits restricted diffusion
- Acute cerebral hyperemia
- Status epilepticus causes transient gyral edema and enhancement
- Gliomatosis cerebri involves more than one lobe

MANAGEMENT

Strict blood pressure control and correction of potential offending agents.

Cortical Laminar Necrosis

Occurs in cardiac arrest, under hypoxemic and hypoglycemic conditions, due to necrosis of neurons in the cortex of the brain. Cortical layers 3, 4, and 5, primary visual cortex and perirolandic region, are selectively prone to metabolic stress.

CLINICAL

Focal neurological deficits due to cerebral hypoperfusion, hypoxia, severe anemia, status epilepticus, carbon monoxide poisoning.

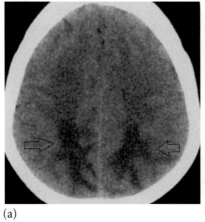
(a)

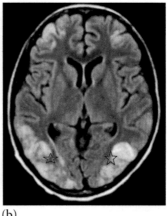
(b)

Figure 2.23 (a and b) Findings of PRES.

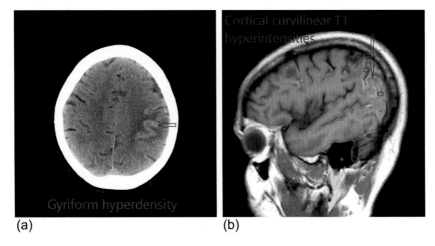
(a)   (b)

Figure 2.24 (a and b) Cortical laminar necrosis.

IMAGING

- CT – gyriform hyperattenuation in the affected cortex, followed by gyral enhancement
- MRI – cortical T1 hyperintensities in a curvilinear pattern, usually after three to four days of a stroke, becoming prominent at around two to four weeks and may fade over 3–4 months
- Cortical enhancement after 2–3 weeks, which persists for a few months
- T2WI – iso- to hyperintense signal. GRE is normal, as no hemorrhage or calcification is noted
- DWI – restricted diffusion

MANAGEMENT

Treatment of the underlying cause.

ANCILLARY

High signal on T1WI is as a result of coagulation necrosis and the accumulation of denatured proteins in dying cells or lipid-laden macrophages.

Fetal Origin of Posterior Cerebral Artery (PCA)

Normal variant in which the dominant supply to occipital lobes is from the internal carotid artery.

- Posterior communicating artery is larger than the ipsilateral P1 segment of the PCA
- Associated with hypoplastic/absent P1 segment of the PCA
- If bilateral, the basilar artery is smaller than normal

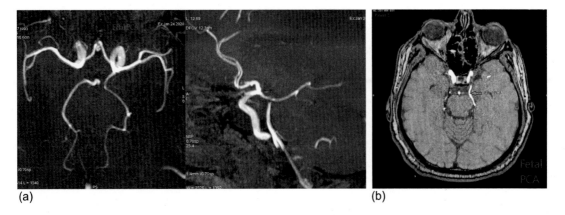
(a)   (b)

Figure 2.25 (a and b) Fetal origin of PCA.

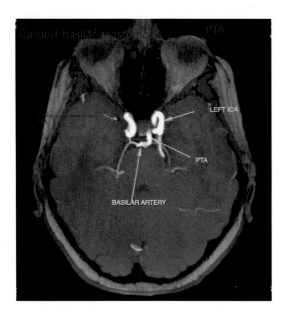

Figure 2.26 PTA.

- PCoM lies superolateral to the 3rd cranial nerve (normally PCoM lies superomedial to the oculomotor nerve)

Persistent Trigeminal Artery (PTA)

- It courses posteromedially from the ICA and anastomoses with the distal basilar artery

- Usually associated with small PComA, vertebral and basilar artery caudal to the anastomoses, and with a high incidence of intracranial aneurysms/vascular malformations
- The presence of PTA in a medial or intrasellar location prior to transsphenoidal surgery for pituitary adenoma is crucial to the report, as an accidental transection of the artery may result in life-threatening hemorrhage
- Neurovascular compression syndrome (trigeminal neuralgia) may result by compression of the PTA

SUGGESTED READING

de Lucas, EM, Sánchez, E, Gutiérrez, A, Mandly, AG, Ruiz, E, Fernández Flórez, A, Izquierdo, J, Arnáiz, J, Piedra, T, Valle, N, Bañales, I, Quintana, F. CT protocol for acute strokes: Tips and tricks for general radiologists. *Radiographics* 2008;28(6):1673–1687.

Dimmick, SJ, Faulder, KC. Normal variants of the cerebral circulation at multidetector CT angiography. *Radiographics* 2009;29(4):1027–1043.

Osborn, AG, Salzman, KL, Jhaveri, MD, Barkovich, AJ. *Diagnostic Imaging: Brain.* Elsevier Health Sciences; 2015.

3

Intracranial Hemorrhage (ICH)

PERINATAL HEMORRHAGE

PRETERM INFANTS

Germinal Matrix Hemorrhage (GMH)

The germinal matrix is a region of thin-walled veins and actively proliferating cells in the subependymal layer of the lateral ventricles. It usually involutes by 34–36 weeks of gestation and has entirely migrated by 40 weeks. GMH is the most common lesion in high-risk low-birth-weight infants, due to hypoxic-ischemic injury to the deep vascular watershed zone in the developing fetus.

IMAGING

Grade 1: Hemorrhage confined to one or both germinal matrices.
Grade 2: Hemorrhage rupture into normal-sized ventricles.
Grade 3: Intraventricular hemorrhage with hydrocephalus.
Grade 4: Extension of hemorrhage into the adjacent white matter of the hemispheres.

TERM INFANTS

ICH in term infants is usually due to traumatic delivery or HIE.

Traumatic Extracranial Hemorrhage

- *Subgaleal hemorrhage* lies under the occipito-frontal galea aponeurotica
- *Caput succedaneum* refers to cutaneous hemorrhagic edema
- *Cephalhematoma* refers to traumatic, subperiosteal hemorrhage limited by sutures

Traumatic Intracranial Hemorrhage

The most common locations include:

- Subdural space (usually along the interhemispheric fissure and tentorium cerebelli)
- Subarachnoid cisterns
- Posterior fossa SAH

Non-Traumatic Intracranial Hemorrhage

Hypoxia ischemic injury occurs due to asphyxia and infarction.

ADULTS

- The spectrum of hemorrhagic infarcts may range from petechiae-like hemorrhages to frank parenchymal hematomas. Usually, hemorrhagic transformation of initially ischemic lesions occurs when an occluded vessel recanalizes and ischemic areas are reperfused, following embolus fragmentation and lysis.
- Pseudolaminar cortical necrosis.
- Cerebral arterial embolism.
- Vascular malformations, as explained in Chapter 2.
- Intra-tumoral hematomas.
- Amyloid angiopathy.
- Inflammatory disease and vasculitides, such as infective endocarditis with septic emboli, fungal vasculitis (aspergillosis), and herpes simplex encephalitis.

- Drugs like cocaine, amphetamines and their derivatives, like phenylpropanol-amine (PPA), phencyclidine, ephedrine, and pseudoephedrine.
- Blood dyscrasias and coagulopathies like congenital clotting disorders, vitamin K deficiency, and disseminated intravascular coagulation (DIC), with secondary fibrinolysis.

Intraventricular Hemorrhage (IVH)

It may occur due to:

- Tearing of subependymal veins along the ventricular surface
- Direct extension of intraparenchymal hemorrhage into the ventricular system
- Retrograde flow of SAH into the ventricular system via foramina

There is a high risk of developing hydrocephalus and infection (ependymitis).

SUBDURAL HEMORRHAGE (SDH) VS. EXTRADURAL HEMORRHAGE (EDH) AND CEREBRAL HERNIATION

It is a common complication of ICH, and occurs when the brain, CSF, and vessels are shifted from one compartment to another, causing loss of brainstem functions. It may also lead to occlusion of blood vessels, hemorrhagic infarcts, and diffuse cerebral edema, adding to the mass effect.

Various types of cerebral herniation include:

1) *Subfalcine herniation* (cingulate herniation): Displacement of brain tissue under the cerebral falx. It results in compression of the ipsilateral ventricle, dilatation of the contralateral ventricle and shifting of the ipsilateral ACA and the subependymal veins across the midline.
2) *Uncal herniation* (downward transtentorial herniation): Medial part of the temporal lobe is pushed down toward the cerebellum. It results in effacement of the ipsilateral suprasellar cistern, basal cisterns, and enlargement of the ipsilateral cerebellopontine angle cistern, along with the inferomedial displacement of the anterior choroidal, PCom, and posterior cerebral arteries in severe cases. It may also result in midbrain hemorrhage (Duret hemorrhage).
3) *Ascending transtentorial herniation*: Less common; upward herniation of vermis and cerebellar hemispheres through the tentorial incisura.
4) *Transalar (transsphenoidal) herniation*.
5) *Tonsillar herniation*: Downward displacement and herniation of the cerebellar tonsils at the level of the foramen magnum.

Other sequelae of trauma include pneumocephalus, encephalomalacia, CSF leaks, and cranial nerve injuries.

Table 3.1 Differentiation between SDH and EDH

	Subdural Hemorrhage	Extradural Hemorrhage
Clinical history	Headache, altered mental status. Consciousness reduces with increasing mass effect	Lucid interval is seen (injury followed by regaining of consciousness and loss of consciousness over the next few hours)
Etiology	Most common factor is non-accidental injury in infants, accidental trauma in young adults, and falls in alcoholics and the elderly age group	Trauma. Usually associated with skull fracture
Source	Usually venous due to tearing of bridging veins, which extend to dural sinuses	Usually arterial in origin (injury to the middle meningeal artery, a branch of the maxillary artery)
Imaging features	Crescentic, concave-shaped collection	Lentiform, biconvex collection
	Crosses sutures	Do not cross sutures
Management	Depends on the extent of the hematoma and clinical condition of the patient	Immediate evacuation

Table 3.2 Appearance of Hematoma on Computed Tomography and Magnetic Resonance Imaging as Per Its Stage

Stage/Age	Hemoglobin Stage	Edema	CT	T1WI	T2/FLAIR	GRE
Hyperacute (4-6 hours)	Oxyhemoglobin	Mild peripheral edema	Hyperdense	Isointense to gray matter	Hyperintense	Hypointense
Acute (7 hours to 2 days)	Deoxyhemoglobin	Marked edema	Hyperdense	Iso- to hypointense	Hypointense	Hypointense
Early subacute (2–7 days)	Intracellular methemoglobin	Edema persists	Hyperdense	Hyperintense rim with isointense center	Hypointense/variable	Hypointense
Late subacute (1–4 weeks)	Extracellular methemoglobin	Edema subsides and mass effect also reduces	Isodense	Hyperintense	Hyperintense	Hyperintense
Chronic (months to years)	Hemosiderin and ferritin	Edema disappears	Hypodense	Iso- to hypointense (hyperintense if rebleed)	Hypointense	Hyperintense core surrounded by hypointense rim

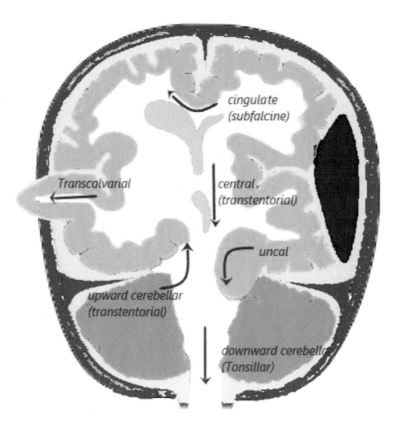

Figure 3.1 Various types of cerebral herniation.

CASE STUDIES

Subdural Hemorrhage (SDH)

Collection of blood in the subdural space between the dura and the arachnoid mater of the meninges.

CLINICAL

Reduced consciousness, history of a trivial fall.

IMAGING

- SDH is generally a crescent-shaped extra-axial collection, hyperdense in the acute stage, with density varying with age of the clot and protein degradation. Occasionally, in patients with anemia and coagulopathies, acute hematomas may be isodense in attenuation.
- Bilateral subacute hematomas are isodense and challenging to diagnose.
- When the hemorrhage is small, the abnormality on a CT scan may be very subtle. Therefore, always look for asymmetries and the presence of an obliterated gyri sulci pattern.

- Small, subdural hematomas may be obscured by volume averaging with adjacent bony structures and are easily delineated in CT on subdural window (wide window –window width WW 130 and window level WL of 30). Coronal reformations should also be included in a trauma protocol for better diagnosis.
- Rebleeding – evolution of SDH results in a heterogeneous motley of fresh blood and partially liquified hematoma (hematocrit effect).
- Chronic SDH – isointense on T1W, hyperintense on T2/FLAIR, with enhancement of neo-membranes.

DDs

- Extradural hematoma
- BESSI – no mass effect (see page 99)
- Subdural hygromas – difficult to differentiate from chronic SDH, exhibiting similar CSF-density hematoma
- Subdural empyemas – peripheral enhancement, along with clinical symptoms of fever and weakness

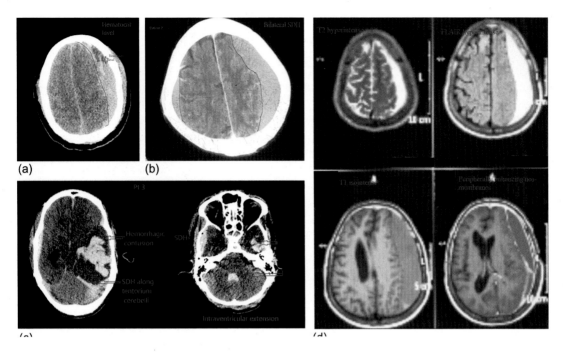

Figure 3.2 (a) Hematocrit effect of SDH, (b) bilateral SDH, (c) SDH along the tentorium cerebelli and the temporal lobe in a patient with hemorrhagic contusion, and (d) imaging findings of SDH on various MRI sequences.

MANAGEMENT

Symptomatic hematomas require surgical evacuation (craniotomy/burr hole).

Epidural Hemorrhage

Collection in the epidural space between the dura mater and the inner table of the skull.

CLINICAL

Patient may regain consciousness (lucid interval) after an episode of traumatic injury till the time the hematoma accumulates and exerts mass effect on the adjacent brain tissue or structures, resulting in the herniation syndrome, that may prove fatal.

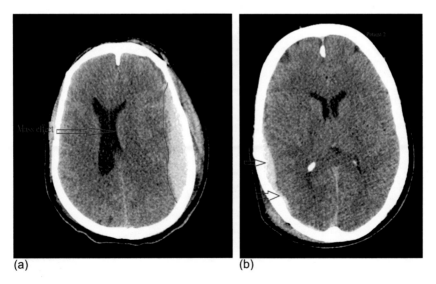

Figure 3.3 (a) Left-sided EDH, (b) right-sided EDH.

IMAGING

- NCCT – biconvex extra-axial collection that displaces the GWM interface away from the calvarium
- Rapid expansion of arterial EDH and active bleed is suggested by the mottled appearance (presence of low attenuation areas within the hyperdense hematoma), due to mixing of hyperacute and acute blood ("swirl sign")
- MRI – displaced dura is seen as a hypointense thin line between the brain and calvarium

DDs

- SDH
- Meningioma – hyperdense, avid, homogeneous contrast enhancement

MANAGEMENT

Surgical evacuation.

Subarachnoid Hemorrhage (SAH)

It may be traumatic or non-traumatic secondary to cerebral aneurysms, arteriovenous malformations, etc. and occur due to injury to arteries or veins coursing through subarachnoid space (SAS). Risk factors include female sex, hypertension, smoking, alcohol use, and cocaine abuse.

CLINICAL

Worst headache ever.

IMAGING

- NCCT – acute stage (initial 48 hours), with abnormal hyperdensity in the SAS (basal cisterns, Sylvian fissure, and interhemispheric fissure), along the cerebral convexities, intraventricular blood fluid levels
- CT angiogram – detects intracranial aneurysms, if any
- MRI – subacute bleed

Lumbar puncture is often required in these patients to show xanthochromia and confirm the diagnosis.

DDs (PSEUDO SAH)

- Diffuse cerebral edema due to pyogenic leptomeningitis, status epilepticus
- Polycythemia
- Extremely premature and unmyelinated brain
- Intrathecally administered contrast and leakage of high-dose intravenous contrast in SASs may mimic SAH on CT scan

MANAGEMENT

It depends on the underlying cause. Monitoring of raised intracranial pressure, drainage for hydrocephalus. Cerebral vasospasm is a crucial complication, resulting in delayed cerebral ischemia

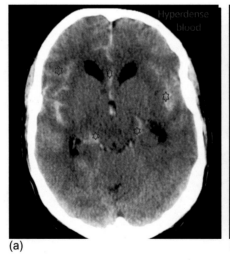
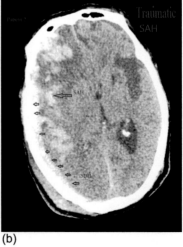

(a)   (b)

Figure 3.4 (a) SAH, (b) SAH with SDH in a patient with traumatic brain injury.

and requires treatment with nimodipine (calcium channel blocker) and endovascular intervention (intra-arterial delivery of vasodilating agents and balloon angioplasty).

Hemorrhagic Parenchymal Contusions

They occur commonly due to injury to arteries or veins, as a result of trauma. The most common sites include the anterior and posterior temporal lobes and the inferior frontal lobes, which are usually adjacent to the bony structure of the skull.

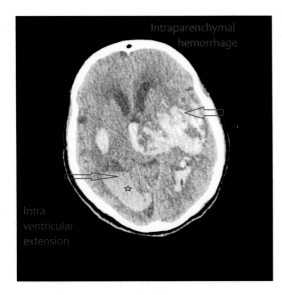

Figure 3.5 Hemorrhagic, intraparenchymal contusion with intraventricular extension.

IMAGING

- NCCT – high-attenuation lesion within the brain parenchyma.
- MRI, especially the GRE sequences, are better at delineating even the small focal hemorrhagic contusions. Traumatic cerebral microhemorrhages are multiple tiny foci of contusions, usually centered in the white matter/GWM junction. They are generally occult on head CT, but are seen as hypointense foci with blooming on SWI/GRE sequences.

DDs

- Trauma
- Intratumoral bleed

MANAGEMENT

Small contusions require proper monitoring as they may expand to sizable intraparenchymal hemorrhage with mass effect in a short period, mandating emergent evacuation or neurosurgical decompression.

Hypertensive Hemorrhage

Hypertensive hemorrhage usually affects elderly hypertensive patients and is found particularly in areas supplied by penetrating branches of the middle cerebral and basilar arteries, preferentially involving putamen, external capsule, thalamus, pons, and cerebellum (near the dentate nucleus).

CLINICAL

Headache, seizures, visual disturbances, focal neurological signs, altered mental status. Common

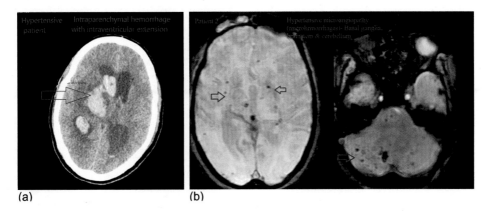

(a) (b)

Figure 3.6 (a) Hypertensive, intraparenchymal hemorrhage with intraventricular extension, (b) hypertensive microangiopathy.

in pregnancy (pre-eclampsia → hypertension + proteinuria) and (eclampsia → pre-eclampsia + convulsions/coma).

IMAGING

- NCCT – intra-axial hyperdense region in the basal ganglia (putamen), cerebellum, or occipital lobes. Large hematomas may result in mass effect and brain herniation. Intraventricular extension of the hemorrhage may also be noted.
- CT angiogram – "spot sign" (active contrast extravasation with pooling, seen as a hyperdense region within the hematoma on delayed scans).

DDs

- Cerebral amyloid angiopathy – a common cause of recurrent ICH in elderly normotensive patients. There are multiple hemorrhagic foci at the corticomedullary junction, with sparing of the basal ganglia and brainstem
- Intratumoral bleed

MANAGEMENT

Serial monitoring for small lesions, surgical decompression/evacuation for larger lesions.

Diffuse Axonal Injury (DAI)

DAI occurs as a result of rotational acceleration/deceleration shearing forces, leading to malalignment of axons and, eventually, to brain edema. Multiple, bilateral, hemorrhagic, and non-hemorrhagic punctate lesions are noted in typical locations at the GWM junction of frontotemporal lobes, corpus callosum (mainly splenium), and brainstem (the dorsolateral midbrain and upper pons).

CLINICAL

Unconsciousness, persistent vegetative state following trauma.

IMAGING

- CT – less sensitive than MRI, but can delineate hyper-attenuated hemorrhagic foci in characteristic locations better than hypodense non-hemorrhagic foci. It is usually associated with cerebral edema and intraventricular hemorrhage.
- GRE/SWI – hemorrhagic lesions showing blooming.
- FLAIR – non-hemorrhagic lesions are punctate and hyperintense.

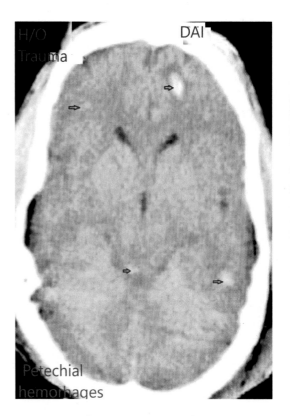

Figure 3.7 Diffuse axonal injury.

- DWI – restricted diffusion, especially in the posterior corpus callosum.

DDs

- Cortical contusions typically involve the cortex and are associated with SDH and SAH
- Cerebral amyloid angiopathy
- Hemorrhagic metastasis
- Multiple cavernomas
- Cerebral fat emboli in a patient with sickle cell anemia or long bone fracture

MANAGEMENT

Prognosis is poor, and management aims to reduce edema by steroids, apart from supportive treatment and long-term rehabilitation.

Non-Accidental Injury (NAI) (Battered Child Syndrome, Shaken Infant Syndrome)

Children, especially under two years, presenting with multiple injuries and inconsistent/suspicious

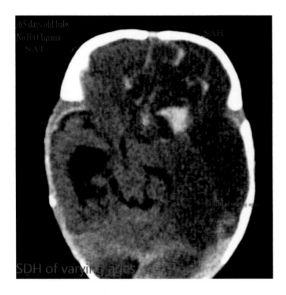

Figure 3.8 SDH of varying ages in an infant (NAI).

history by parents/guardians, should be considered as NAI until proved otherwise.

IMAGING

- Skeletal survey to detect other fractures like:
  - Metaphyseal fractures (bucket handle/corner fractures)
  - Posterior and lateral rib fractures
  - Non-parietal skull fractures (mostly occipital bones and fractures crossing the sutures)
  - Fracture of sternum, scapula, spinous processes
  - Bilateral fractures of different ages are typical of NAI
- Subdural hematomas, especially interhemispheric SDH

- Visceral perforation or hematoma, liver, and pancreatic injuries
- Retinal hemorrhages

DDs

- Osteogenesis imperfecta – look for other features, like bowing of bones, osteopenia, and the presence of Wormian bones
- Accidental injury

Depressed Skull Fracture

High-energy impact to the skull results in inward folding of skull vault into the cerebral parenchyma, the most common site being the frontoparietal region. Depending on the number of pieces of bones, the fracture can be a hinged door (one piece) or comminuted (multiple pieces).

IMAGING

- NCCT (bone window) – delineates the fracture and associated soft tissue swelling external to the site of fracture
- Soft tissue window – demonstrates associated intracranial hemorrhage, pneumocephalus, and cerebral edema

DDs

- Sutures are symmetrical and well corticated

MANAGEMENT

Elevation of depressed fragments.

ANCILLARY

Other types of fractures include:

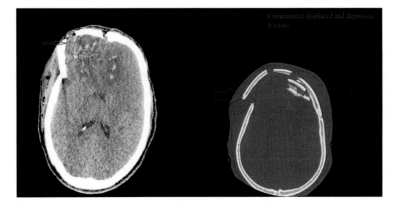

Figure 3.9 Depressed fracture of skull.

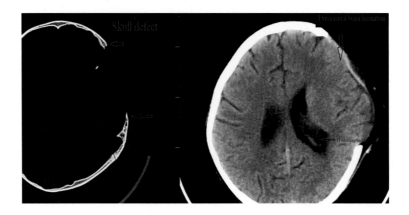

Figure 3.10 Leptomeningeal cyst.

- Linear fracture – fracture fragments are not displaced
- Growing skull fracture
- Ping pong fracture – synonymous with greenstick fracture of long bones, it occurs in children as a result of a fall, when the skull hits the edge of a hard, blunt object
- Diastatic fracture – fracture line traverses the sutures and leads to sutural widening

Leptomeningeal Cyst (Growing Skull Fracture)

Usually occurs in children after severe head trauma, resulting in dural tear and herniation of the brain and meninges.

CLINICAL

Seizures, growing scalp mass.

IMAGING

CT and MRI:

- Skull defect with scalloped edges and extracranial brain herniation
- Encephalomalacic changes
- Hydrocephalus

DDs

Calvarial metastasis.

MANAGEMENT

Surgery.

SUGGESTED READING

Adam, A. *Grainger & Allison's Diagnostic Radiology: A Textbook of Medical Imaging.* Churchill Livingstone; 2008.

Edward Sellon, DH. *Radiology for Medical Finals: A Case Based Guide.* 1st ed. Boca Raton, FL: Taylor & Francis, CRC Press; 2018.

Osborn, AG, Salzman, KL, Jhaveri, MD, Barkovich, AJ. *Diagnostic Imaging: Brain.* Elsevier Health Sciences; 2015.

Watson, N, Watson, NA, Jones, H. *Chapman & Nakielny's Guide to Radiological Procedures.* Elsevier; 2018.

4

Radiology of Brain Tumors

ANALYTICAL APPROACH

Imaging diagnosis of brain neoplasms is based on:

- Location of lesion (supra- *vs.* infratentorial/intra- *vs.* extra-axial)
- Morphological analysis (size, margins, enhancement pattern)
- Associated secondary changes, like edema, calcification, hemorrhage, etc.

AGE DISTRIBUTION

Common tumors of the pediatric age group are choroid plexus papillomas, teratomas, medulloblastoma, craniopharyngiomas, ependymomas, and metastases from neuroblastoma.

Tumors frequently afflicting adults include metastases, astrocytomas, glioblastoma multiforme, meningiomas, oligodendrogliomas, pituitary adenomas, and schwannomas.

LOCATION

See Table 4.1.

EDEMA

Peritumoral edema is the non-enhancing area of abnormality surrounding the enhancing tumor core.

In metastatic brain tumors and non-infiltrative primary tumors, such as meningiomas, peritumoral edema corresponds to vasogenic edema, where there is leakage of plasma fluid from altered tumor capillaries, but no tumor cells are present.

In gliomas, the peritumoral edema corresponds to infiltrative edema, as, apart from vasogenic edema, the infiltrating tumor cells behind the blood–brain barrier (BBB) invade along the white matter tracts.

MIDLINE CROSSING LESIONS

- Glioblastoma multiforme (GBM) – by infiltrating the white matter tracts of the corpus callosum
- Lymphoma is usually located near the midline
- Meningioma (an extra-axial tumor) – along the meninges to the contralateral side
- Radiation necrosis
- Epidermoid cysts – *via* the subarachnoid space
- Multiple sclerosis

MULTIFOCAL/MULTIPLE TUMORS

- Metastatic disease
- Lymphomas
- Multicentric GBM
- Gliomatosis cerebri
- Phakomatosis like neurofibromatosis type II
- Seeding metastases as in medulloblastomas (PNET-MB)

Subarachnoid seeding is seen as tumoral nodules along with the brain and spinal cord, e.g., primitive neuroectodermal tumors (PNET), like medulloblastoma and pineoblastoma, ependymoma, choroid plexus papilloma, GBM, and lymphoma.

Cortical-based tumors, like oligodendroglioma, ganglioglioma, and dysembryoplastic neuroepithelial tumor (DNET), usually present with complex seizures.

Table 4.1 Differentiation between Extra-Axial and Intra-Axial Lesions

Finding	Extra-Axial	Intra-Axial
Attachment to dura/bone	Contiguous	Not attached unless advanced
Cortical displacement	Away from bone	Toward the dura/bone
Feeding vessels	Dural arteries	Pial arteries
Local bony changes	Common	Uncommon
Subarachnoid cistern	Widened	Effaced
Examples	Meningioma, schwannoma	Metastasis, astrocytoma

Table 4.2 Comparison of Cytotoxic and Vasogenic Edema

Cytotoxic Edema	Vasogenic Edema
Failure of the energy pump at the cell membrane level results in sodium influx and intracellular swelling	Disturbance of vascular permeability enables the indiscriminate escape of plasma fluid and protein
Marked decrease in extracellular space	Increase in extracellular space volume
Implies permanent cellular damage (irreversible)	Implies reactive changes (reversible)
Acute infarct	GBM

SIGNAL CHARACTERISTICS

Tumors with High Density on CT Scan

- Colloid cyst
- Lymphoma
- Medulloblastoma

Fat

- CT (–100 HU) – low density
- MR – high signal intensity on both T1WI and T2WI
- Fat-suppression sequences like STIR – low signal intensity of fat
- STIR differentiates hyperintense subacute hematoma, melanin, and slow flow from fat on T1WI

Chemical shift artifact (alternating bands of high and low signal on the boundaries of a lesion seen only in the frequency encoding direction) indicates the presence of fat. Intratumoral fat is seen in lipomas, dermoid cysts, and teratomas.

Calcification

- CT – high density.
- MRI – hypointense on T1, T2WI, and GRE; challenging to differentiate from hemorrhage

sometimes. SWI (susceptibility-weighted imaging) differentiates hemorrhage from calcifications.

Usually, tumors are hypointense on T1WI and hyperintense on T2WI due to high water content. Exceptions to this rule suggest a specific type of tumor.

Low SI on T2WI

- Dense and hypercellular tumors with a high nuclear-cytoplasmic ratio like CNS lymphoma and medulloblastoma (also hyperdense on CT)
- Calcified tumors
- Tumors with hemosiderin content (signal drop due to paramagnetic effects)
- Tumors with mucinous/proteinaceous material like a colloid cyst
- Tumors with flow voids (suggesting the presence of vessels or flow within a lesion) like hemangioblastomas, though also noted in nontumorous lesions like vascular malformations

High Signal Intensity on T1

- Contrast enhancement
- Fat, as in lipoma, dermoid cyst
- High protein/mucin content, as in colloid cyst

- Methemoglobin, as in hemorrhage (subacute) and thrombosed aneurysm
- Melanin (melanoma metastases)
- Paramagnetic cations like copper, manganese
- Slow flow

ENHANCEMENT PATTERN

The triple-layered BBB, with tight endothelial junctions in the brain, maintains a consistent internal milieu. The contrast will not leak into the brain unless this barrier is damaged.

- CNS tumor destroys the BBB – enhancement present.
- Extra-axial tumors (not derived from brain tissue) – do not have a BBB – homogeneous enhancement. BBB is absent in the pituitary, choroid plexus, and pineal regions.
- Non-tumoral lesions (like infections, demyelinating diseases (MS) and infarctions) – break down the BBB – enhancement present and may simulate a brain tumor.

Little/No Enhancement

- Low-grade astrocytomas
- Cystic non-tumoral lesions, like a dermoid cyst, epidermoid, or arachnoid cyst

Ring Enhancement

M – Metastases – known primary, multiplicity
A – Abscess – MRS
G – GBM (glioblastoma multiforme) – MRS, perfusion study
I – Infarct (subacute phase) – territorial distribution
C – Contusion/hematoma (resolving) – history of trauma, hemosiderin rim
D – Demyelinating lesion (MS – with an incomplete rim of enhancement)
R – Radiation necrosis – specific history

RECENT ADDITIONS TO THE WHO CLASSIFICATION OF TUMORS

MVNT (Multinodular Vacuolating Neuronal Tumor) of the Cerebrum

This benign lesion was described in the WHO CNS Tumors in 2016. Patients usually present with seizures, and the lesion is found predominantly in the temporal lobe, involving the cortex and the superficial white matter.

IMAGING

- CT – usually normal unless the lesion is large
- MRI – non-enhancing lesion with low to intermediate SI on T1 WI and hyperintense on T2/FLAIR sequences without any mass effect or edema and calcifications
  - No restricted diffusion

DDs

- DNET

Diffuse Leptomeningeal Glioneuronal Tumor

It is seen mainly in children. Diffuse, plaque-like, and enhancing the subarachnoid tumor generally along the spinal cord, with frequent involvement of the posterior fossa, brainstem, and basilar cisterns, as well as Sylvian and interhemispheric fissures. Small cystic or nodular T2-hyperintense lesions can be seen superficially along the parenchymal surface, representing expansion and fibrosis of subarachnoid spaces.

Tumor Mimics

Many non-tumorous lesions can simulate a brain tumor.

- Abscesses
- Multiple sclerosis (tumefactive)
- Aneurysm, especially in parasellar region

Imaging

Apart from T1, T2, FLAIR sequences.

DWI (Diffusion-Weighted Imaging)

DWI generates images that are based on the molecular motion of water, which is altered by the disease.

Limitations

1) Malignancy with cystic/necrotic component shows high ADC due to lack of restriction
2) If the rim of the lesion is too thin for correct ROI placement

Table 4.3 Differentiation between Malignant and Benign Lesions on DWI

Malignant Lesions	Benign Lesions
Tightly packed cells leading to inhibition of effective movement of water molecules	High water mobility, increased diffusion process
Restricted diffusion (increased SI on DWI)	Reduced SI on DWI
Low ADC value	High ADC value

3) Nonfocal masses/diffuse tumor spread may not be categorized.
4) Carcinomas with excessive increased SI on T2 (mucinous tumors) → misleading ADC value due to differential cell packing

DWI is used to assess:

- Tumor grade and cellularity
- Postoperative injury
- Peritumoral edema
- Integrity of white matter tracts.

SWI (Susceptibility-Weighted Imaging)

High-resolution T2 gradient echo (GRE) sequence, is highly sensitive to magnetic susceptibility effects from blood products or mineralization. This sequence is useful to differentiate between hemorrhage and calcification in tumors, both of which appear dark on magnitude images. On filtered phase images, paramagnetic blood products appear dark, and diamagnetic calcium appears bright.

DTI (Diffusion Tensor Imaging)

DTI provides a 3-D representation of white matter integrity to determine whether there is tumor invasion, displacement, disruption, infiltration of the adjacent white matter tracts, and helps as a non-invasive tool, providing an intraoperative guide to avoiding injury to the corticospinal tract during tumor resection.

Two formats:

1) FA (fractional anisotropy) maps and directionally encoded color maps
2) 3-D tractography

MRS (MR Spectroscopy)

A non-invasive technique to determine the molecular metabolites within the body and for early detection of ailments, since, in many pathological processes, metabolic changes precede anatomical changes during disease progression and treatment.

The most recognizable metabolite peaks on long-echo ^{1}H-MRS include:

- *NAA (N- acetyl aspartate) major upfield peak* at 2.02 ppm (parts per million) (a marker of neuronal viability). Reduced in tumors, demyelination, infarcts, increased in Canavan's disease.
- *Choline peak* at 3.22 ppm (cell membrane turnover marker).
- *Creatine peak* at 3.02 ppm (energy marker; reflects normal cellular metabolism).
- *Lactate peak* at 1.33 ppm (may be seen as a doublet; indicates hypoxia).
- *Lipid peaks* at 0.9–1.3 ppm (broad peaks; a marker of necrosis).
- *Myo-inositol (MI) peak* at 3.5 ppm. (reflects astrocyte integrity).
- *Taurine peak* at 3.4 ppm is suggestive of primitive neuroectodermal tumors, particularly in children.

1) Brain tumors
   - Increased choline and choline/creatine ratio
   - Reduced NAA
2) Differentiating between radiation necrosis and tumor recurrence
   - Choline increased in recurrence while reduced in necrosis

Hence, MRS is used in both the diagnosis and evaluation of treatment response of brain tumors.

Perfusion Imaging

Perfusion imaging measures the degree of tumor angiogenesis and capillary permeability, both of which are important biological markers of malignancy, grading, and prognosis, and for differentiating radiation necrosis from tumor recurrence.

Can be used to measure four perfusion parameters:

- *CBV (cerebral blood volume)* – the volume of blood per unit of brain tissue (4–5 ml/ 100 g)
- *CBF (cerebral blood flow)* – the volume of blood flow per unit of brain tissue per minute (50–60 ml/100 g/min)
- *MTT (mean transit time)* – time difference between arterial inflow and venous outflow
  - MTT = CBV/CBF
- *Time to peak enhancement* – time from beginning of contrast material injection to the maximum concentration of contrast material within ROI

In gliomas, the perfusion curve returns to normal in comparison to tumors with leaky capillaries (metastasis, extra-axial tumors, and choroid plexus tumors) in which the perfusion curve does not return to the baseline.

Dynamic Contrast Enhancement (DCE) measures volume transfer constant, a measure of permeability, which is directly proportional to grade, progression, and recurrence of the tumor.

The primary variable measured in Dynamic Susceptibility Contrast (DSC) perfusion technique is relative CBV (rCBV), directly proportional to grade, progression, and recurrence of the tumor. The value is high in pilocytic astrocytomas (WHO grade I astrocytoma with homogeneous vascular hyperplasia), glioblastoma multiforme (WHO grade IV astrocytoma with heterogeneous vascular hyperplasia), non-astrocytic gliomas like oligodendrogliomas (low grade but known for its neoangiogenic vessels – "chicken-wire" vasculature).

CBF is mainly measured by Arterial Spin Labelling (ASL), a non-contrast method to assess tumor grading and progression.

PET-CT

Provides both anatomical and functional information in a single imaging study.

FDG (fluorodeoxyglucose) images the glucose metabolic rate. Malignant tumor cells with high metabolic activity use more glucose than normal cells.

Wait for 60–80 minutes after intravenous FDG, before taking the scan.

CT takes 60–70 seconds followed by a PET scan that takes 30–45 minutes.

Used for staging (upstaging and downstaging), restaging, assessment of therapy response, follow-up evaluation and detection of recurrence.

High glucose metabolism in recurrent brain glioma differentiates it from post-radiotherapy changes.

High uptake of ^{11}C-methionine by PET (reflects cellular amino acid uptake) is suggestive of high-grade glioma and poor survival. The use of ^{11}C-methionine PET also aids in differentiating tumoral from non-tumoral intracranial bleed, based on an increased ^{11}C-methionine concentration in tumoral bleed.

BOLD (Blood Oxygen Level-Dependent) Imaging

This refers to the contrast effect between oxygenated and deoxygenated hemoglobin that forms the technical basis of functional MRI. Deoxygenated hemoglobin, with its paramagnetic effect, results in a slight signal loss in susceptibility-sensitive sequences, whereas oxygenated hemoglobin, with its diamagnetic characteristics, causes no signal loss in these sequences. It can be applied to demonstrate eloquent brain areas before surgery, as well as functional plasticity of the brain after therapy.

Long-Term Complications of Chemo-/Radiotherapy

- Pseudoprogression is an inflammatory response marked by a transient increase in contrast enhancement and edema upon completion of chemoradiotherapy, but reveals subsequent stabilization or improvement of contrast enhancement at follow-up MRI
- Symmetric white matter signal abnormality represents gradual demyelination, gliosis, and vascular injury, resulting in progressive neurocognitive decline and disordered white matter diffusion
- Scattered foci of susceptibility (microhemorrhages) on SWI may be noticed years later
- Diffuse necrotizing leukoencephalopathy
- Stroke-like Migraine Attacks After Radiation Therapy (SMART) syndrome may ensue rarely. It demonstrates abnormal cortical enhancement but is self-limited and resolves within a few weeks
- Radiation-associated tumors like meningioma, gliomas, and sarcomas

CLASSIFICATION

Supratentorial Tumors

PRIMARY BRAIN TUMORS

Glial Tumors

- *Astrocytoma*
  - Low-grade astrocytoma (Kernohan grade 1,2)
  - Pilocytic astrocytoma
  - Pleomorphic xanthoastrocytoma (PXA)
  - Subependymal giant cell astrocytoma (SEGA)
  - Anaplastic astrocytoma (Kernohan grade 3)
  - Glioblastoma multiforme (Kernohan grade 4)
  - Gliosarcoma
- *Oligodendroglioma*
- *Ependymal tumors*
  - Ependymoma
  - Myxopapillary ependymoma
- *Choroid plexus tumors*
  - Choroid plexus papilloma (CPP)
  - Choroid plexus carcinoma (CPC)

Non-Glial Tumors

- Ganglioglioma/gangliocytoma
- Central neurocytoma
- DNETs (Dysplastic Neuroepithelial Tumors)
- Esthesioneuroblastoma (ENB)
- Lhermitte-Duclos disease (LDD)

HEMATOPOIETIC TUMORS

- Lymphoma
- Leukemia
- Plasmacytoma

Sellar and Suprasellar Tumors

- Adenomas
- Craniopharyngioma

MENINGEAL AND MESENCHYMAL TUMORS

- Meningioma
- Hemangiopericytoma
- Non-meningiotheliomatous mesenchymal tumors
- Hemangioblastoma

Embryonal Tumors

- Primitive neuroectodermal tumor (PNET)
- Neuroblastoma
- Retinoblastoma

PINEAL REGION TUMORS

Germ Cell Tumors (GCTs)

- Germinoma
- Embryonal cell carcinoma
- Yolk sac tumor
- Choriocarcinoma
- Teratoma

Pineal Cell Tumors

Nerve Tumors

- Neurofibromas
- Schwannomas
- Malignant peripheral nerve sheath tumor (MPNST)

Cysts and Tumor Mimics

- Dermoid
- Epidermoid
- Colloid cyst
- Rathke cleft cyst
- Neuroglial cysts, lipomas, hamartomas

MISCELLANEOUS

- Paragangliomas
- Chordomas

Secondary Brain Tumors (Metastasis)

- Leptomeningeal metastasis
- Dural metastasis
- Calvarial metastasis
- Parenchymal metastasis

Infratentorial Tumors

Cerebellum

- Medulloastrocytoma
- Ependymoma
- Hemangioblastoma
- Rhabdoid tumor
- Metastasis
- Pilocytic astrocytoma

Brainstem

- Brainstem glioma
- PNET
- Ganglioglioma

4th Ventricle

- Medulloblastoma
- Ependymoma

- Subependymoma
- Epidermoid
- Choroid plexus papilloma

Cerebello-Pontine Angle (CPA) and Internal Auditory Canal (IAC)

- Schwannoma
- Epidermoid
- Meningiomas
- Metastasis

CASE STUDIES

Glioblastoma Multiforme

One of the most common adult primary intracranial neoplasms, this aggressive WHO grade IV astrocytoma is usually multifocal and metacentric, resistant to therapy, and has a poor prognosis. It can spread along the white matter tracts of corpus callosum to involve the contralateral hemisphere ("butterfly pattern"). It can be primary (arise *de novo*) or secondary (arise from a pre-existing low-grade diffuse astrocytoma).

CLINICAL

Symptoms of raised intracranial tension, focal neurological deficits, seizures.

IMAGING

- CT – heterogeneously hypodense (due to necrotic center), irregularly thick-marginated intra-axial lesion with marked surrounding edema and mass effect. It may be associated with hemorrhage and calcification.
- CECT – intense heterogeneous ring enhancement.
- MRI – the lesion is hypointense on T1, hyperintense on T2 and FLAIR, with central heterogeneities due to necrosis and intratumoral hemorrhage. It is associated with intense vasogenic edema and mass effect.
- CE-MRI – irregular peripheral enhancement.
- GRE/SWI – blooming (blood products).

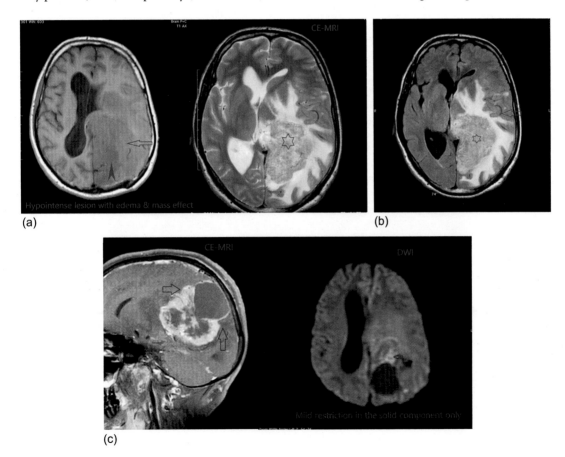

Figure 4.1 (a–c) Imaging findings of GBM.

- DWI – restricted diffusion with high signal in the solid component of the tumor. High ADC values in the non-enhancing necrotic component of the tumor.
- MR perfusion – high rCBV.
- MRS – increased choline, lipids, and lactate with reduced NAA.
- PET – abnormally high metabolism due to the accumulation of FDG.

DDs

- Cerebral metastasis – centered on gray–white matter junction and spare the overlying cortex.
- Primary CNS lymphoma in AIDS patients, as, in this setting, central necrosis is more common; otherwise, lymphoma is usually homogeneously enhancing.
- Cerebral abscess – central restricted diffusion and presence of "double rim" sign (two concentric rims – hypointense outer and hyperintense inner rim – on both SWI and T2WI). The rim is usually smooth and complete, in comparison with GBM, in which the rim is irregular and incomplete. MRS will not show elevated choline: creatine ratio.

MANAGEMENT

Biopsy followed by tumor debulking, with postoperative adjuvant radiotherapy and chemotherapy.

Oligodendroglioma

Frequent in middle-aged adults, particularly common in males, with involvement of the frontal lobe.

CLINICAL

Seizures, headache, nausea, vomiting, visual complaints, and focal neurological deficits.

IMAGING

- NCCT – cortical/ subcortical, well-marginated, mixed-density tumor with calcifications.
  - Minimal peritumoral vasogenic edema.
  - Pressure remodeling/ focal thinning of the overlying skull due to its superficial location.
  - Hemorrhage and cystic degeneration rarely.
- CECT –heterogeneous enhancement.
- MRI – the lesion is hypointense on T1W and hyperintense on T2W, with calcifications appearing as areas of signal loss.
- SWI (filtered phase) – differentiates calcifications from hemorrhage.
- CE-MRI – variable enhancement.
- DWI – no restricted diffusion.
- MR perfusion – elevated rCBV ("chicken wire" network of increased vascularity).
- PET (^{11}C-methionine) – hyper-metabolism in most oligodendrogliomas. It helps in differentiating from astrocytomas and in detecting tumor recurrence.

DDs

- Astrocytoma – involve subcortical white matter and deep gray matter, white matter tracts, and may cross the midline.
- Ganglioglioma – partially cystic mass with an enhancing mural nodule. Most frequently involves temporal lobe and is seen in the younger age group.

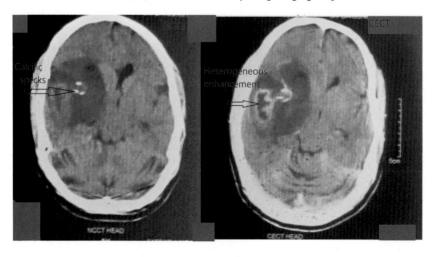

Figure 4.2 Oligodendroglioma on NCCT and CECT.

MANAGEMENT

Surgery, with adjuvant chemo-radiotherapy.

Meningioma

Extra-axial, non-glial neoplasm that originates from the meningocytes or arachnoid cap cells of the meninges. More common in females. Locations can be seen in Figure 4.3f.

CLINICAL

Headache, altered mental status, seizures.

IMAGING

- CT – well-circumscribed, hyperdense mass with broad base toward dura and exhibits "dural tail" sign. May be associated with hyperostosis of underlying bones, calcification, and vasogenic edema.
- CECT – intense homogeneous enhancement.

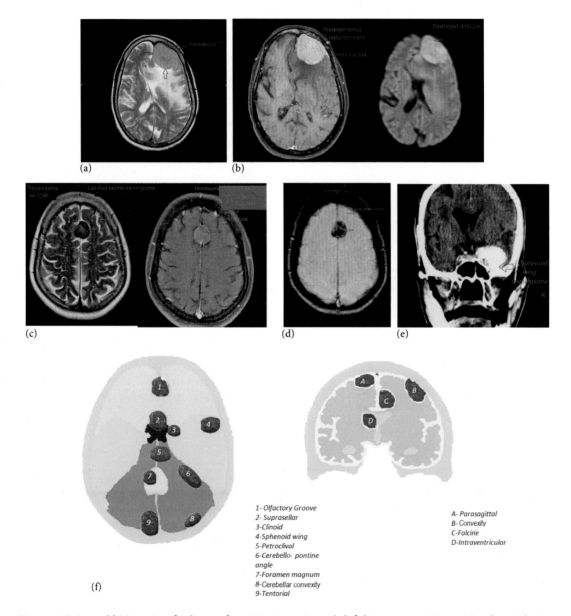

Figure 4.3 (a and b) Imaging findings of meningioma, (c and d) falcine meningioma, (e) sphenoid wing meningioma, (f) common locations of meningioma.

- MRI – isointense to gray matter on T1 and T2 WI.
  - Intense homogeneous post-contrast enhancement.
  - Restricted diffusion.
- MRS – alanine peak.
- Angiography – "mother-in-law" sign, with dense tumor; contrast blush comes early and stays late.
  - "Sunburst" sign due to dual blood supply from meningeal and pial vessels.

LOCATIONS

See Figure 4.3f.

DDs

- Dural metastases – multiple with known primary (breast, prostate)
- Hemangiopericytoma – more lobulated, hypervascular, and locally aggressive tumor with the destruction of overlying bone
- Solitary fibrous tumor of dura: "yin–yang" sign – areas of high and low signal on T2WI, with myoinositol peak on MRS

Few Location-Specific Differentials

- Sella/pituitary macroadenoma – encases the vessels, but no narrowing is seen.
  - Meningioma causes narrowing of vessels along with encasement
- Optic nerve – glioma – optic nerve cannot be seen separately
  - Meningioma – ("tram-track" sign); optic nerve can be seen through the meningioma
  - Intraventricular – xanthogranuloma: T2 shine-through on ADC
  - Meningioma – isointense to gray matter with actual diffusion restriction
- CP angle – schwannoma – extends into internal auditory canal (IAC), causing expansion giving "ice cream cone" appearance
  - Meningioma – usually does not extend into IAC. Even if it spreads, it does not cause expansion

MANAGEMENT

- Surgical excision
- External beam radiation therapy

ANCILLARY

- Meningiomas are estrogen and progesterone sensitive and can increase in size during pregnancy

- Burnt-out meningioma – heavily calcified meningioma
- Radiation-induced meningioma – multiple meningiomas are seen in those exposed to radiation

Cerebello-Pontine Angle (CPA) Schwannoma (Acoustic Neuroma/ Vestibular Schwannoma)

Benign nerve sheath lesions arising from the 8th cranial nerve.

CLINICAL

Sensorineural hearing loss, non-pulsatile tinnitus.

IMAGING

- CT – Expansion and erosion of internal auditory meatus. Extra-axial, heterogeneously enhancing lesion with cystic component but no calcifications.
- MRI
  - Heterogeneously hypointense on T1WI and hyperintense on T2WI with variable enhancement, and adjacent edema and mass effect.
  - The lesion extends into IAM, giving "ice cream cone" appearance.
  - Ipsilateral enlargement of CPA cistern.
  - CSF/vascular cleft between the cerebellum and the mass lesion.
  - Displaced gray–white matter interface around the mass lesion.
  - Brainstem rotated.
  - Compressed 4th ventricle with dilated lateral and 3rd ventricles.
- GRE – foci of intratumoral microhemorrhages.

DDs

- Meningioma – hyperdense, calcifications frequent, does not extend into IAM, homogeneous enhancement
- Epidermoid – restricted diffusion on DWI
- Dolichoectasia/saccular aneurysm of vertebrobasilar artery
- Ependymoma
- Metastasis

MANAGEMENT

Surgical resection.

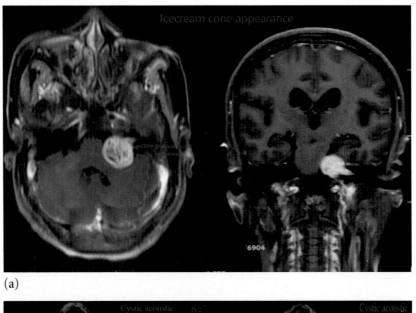

(a)

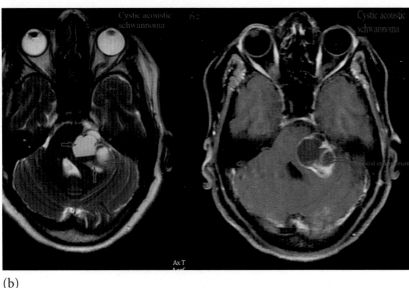

(b)

Figure 4.4 (a) "Ice cream cone" appearance of schwannoma, (b) cystic acoustic schwannoma.

ANCILLARY

CPA cistern lies between the anterolateral surface of the pons and cerebellum and posterior surface of the petrous temporal bone.

Structures within CPA cistern:

- 5th, 7th, 8th cranial nerves
- Superior and anteroinferior cerebellar arteries
- Tributaries of superior petrosal vein

Pituitary Adenoma

- Pituitary microadenoma <10 mm
- Pituitary macroadenoma >10 mm

CLINICAL

Hormonal imbalance, mass effect on adjacent structures (bitemporal hemianopia due to compression of the optic chiasm, cranial nerve deficits due to cavernous sinus invasion).

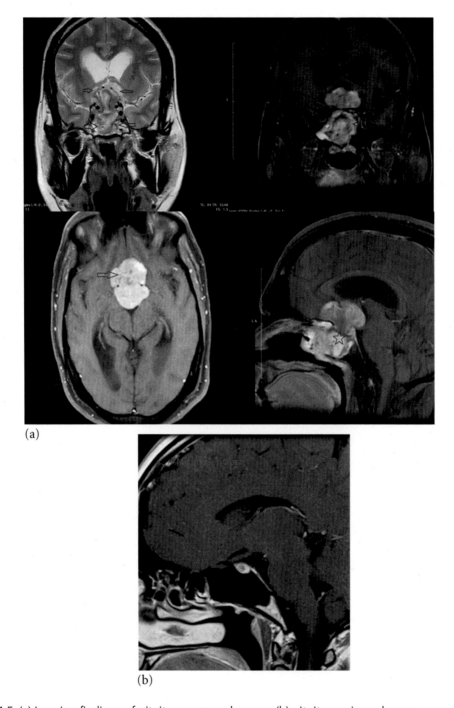

Figure 4.5 (a) Imaging findings of pituitary macroadenoma, (b) pituitary microadenoma.

IMAGING

- NCCT – isodense tumors with attenuation depending on hemorrhage, or cystic degeneration.
- CECT – moderate contrast enhancement.
- MRI – isointense to gray matter on T1W and T2WI, with moderate to intense enhancement of the solid components.
- GRE/SWI – hemorrhagic areas.

- MRI is the superb modality to delineate the involvement of anterior cerebral vessels, cavernous sinus, and optic tract. Blood-fluid levels suggestive of hemorrhage may be demonstrated.

Post-contrast dynamic acquisition – bolus injection of intravenous gadolinium, followed by multiple coronal images of pituitary gland to delineate temporal changes in signal intensity in intrasellar structures.

MICROADENOMAS

- Normal pituitary shows an early and greater degree of enhancement in comparison with adenoma that exhibits less and delayed uptake of contrast.
- Immediately after contrast administration, the signal intensity rises quickly and to a greater degree in the normal pituitary gland than in the microadenoma. Even on dynamic CECT, adenoma appears as a hypodense region within the enhancing gland.
- Within 3–5 minutes of contrast administration, the signal intensity of both the adenoma and the normal pituitary becomes similar.
- Delayed post-contrast images > 20 minutes exhibit slower washout of accumulated contrast, and microadenomas appear hyperintense.

Indirect signs:

- Gland enlargement with the bulge in its outline
- Infundibulum deviation (pituitary stalk tilting)
- Sellar floor asymmetry

MACROADENOMAS

- Sellar expansion with the superior extension of the tumor, above the diaphragmatic sella, gives snowman or figure-of-8 configuration (due to constriction by the diaphragma sella) to adenoma
- Chiasmal displacement
- Sphenoid sinus erosion
- Invasion of the suprasellar cistern
- Cavernous sinus invasion is suggested by encasement of cavernous carotid vessels and delayed enhancing soft tissue lesion in sinus, along with lateral bulging of outer dura
- Solid adenomas show a uniform and early enhancement in comparison to microadenomas due to difference in their blood supply
- PET – intense FDG uptake in macroadenomas

PITUITARY APOPLEXY

Hemorrhage or infarction in pituitary can be spontaneous or in response to bromocriptine therapy for prolactinomas. It is visualized as hyperdense areas on NCCT, bright on T1W (subacute blood) and dark on T2W (acute blood).

DDs

- Pituitary carcinoma – very rare and difficult to distinguish. Look for any CSF seeding.
- Pituitary metastasis – consider if any primary malignancy is known. Bone destruction is more common than remodeling.
- Meningioma – hyperdense with intense uniform enhancement.
- Craniopharyngioma – heterogeneous solid-cystic lesion with calcifications and variable enhancement.
- Optic chiasm glioma – hypo- to isodense, with chiasmal enlargement and retrochiasmal extension; variable enhancement.
- Patent/thrombosed aneurysm.

MANAGEMENT

- Medical treatment with dopaminergic agonists (bromocriptine) for prolactinomas and somatostatin analogs (octreotide) for growth hormone reduction
- Stereotactic radiosurgery
- Transsphenoidal resection of the tumor

ANCILLARY

Adenohypophysis (anterior lobe of the pituitary gland) is isointense on T1 and T2WI. It constitutes pars tuberalis, pars intermedia (Rathke's pouch), and pars distalis. Hormones include growth hormone (GH), adrenocorticotropic hormone (ACTH), thyroid-stimulating hormone (TSH), luteinizing hormone (LH), and prolactin (Prl).

Neurohypophysis (posterior lobe) is bright (hyperintense) on T1 and secretes oxytocin and vasopressin.

Craniopharyngioma

Benign, slow growing, WHO grade I neoplasm, which arises from epithelial remnants in the sellar/suprasellar region (from 3rd ventricle to pituitary gland).

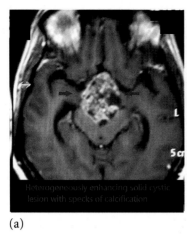 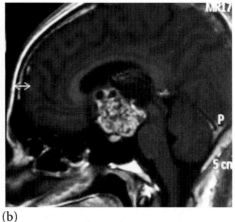

(a)   (b)

Figure 4.6 (a and b) Craniopharyngioma.

CLINICAL

Headache, raised intracranial pressure, and visual symptoms.

IMAGING

There are two histological subtypes, adamantinomatous and papillary types.

DDs

Discussed under "Pituitary Adenoma."

MANAGEMENT

Treatment is usually surgical (transsphenoidal approach) with radiotherapy.

Epidermoid Cyst

Intracranial epidermoid cysts can be congenital or acquired and occur due to the inclusion of ectodermal elements during neural tube closure.

CLINICAL

Headache, cranial nerve deficits, cerebellar symptoms, and seizures.

LOCATION

Cerebello-pontine angle > suprasellar cisterns > 4th ventricle > middle cranial fossa.

IMAGING

- Non-enhancing, CSF density lobulated lesion that fills and expands CSF spaces, insinuating between structures, and encasing adjacent nerves and vessels. It displaces the basilar artery away from the pons.
- MRI – hypointense on TIW and hyperintense on T2W and FLAIR.
- High cholesterol content, if found in the epidermoid cyst(white epidermoid) results in hyperdensity on CT or T1 hyperintensity due to hemorrhage, saponification, or high protein content.

Table 4.4 Comparison of Adamantinomatous and Papillary Types

Adamantinomatous Type	Papillary Type
More common	Less frequent
Predominantly in children, though a second peak may be noted in adults	Exclusively in adults
Calcification is common (peripheral and stippled)	Calcification is rare
Cystic component is common; usually lobulated	Solid component is common, with few cystic areas; usually spherical
Iso- to hyperintense on T1WI and T2WI due to wet keratin nodules (cholesterol-/protein-rich)	Hypointense on T1 and T2WI. No wet keratin
MRS exhibits broad lipid spectrum	No broad lipid spectrum noted

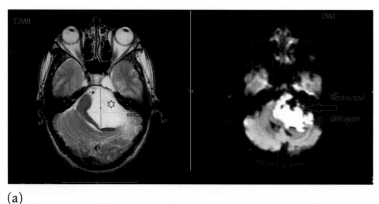

(a)

(b)

Figure 4.7 (a) CPA epidermoid cyst, (b) imaging findings of epidermoid cyst on various sequences.

- DWI – restricted diffusion (hallmark).

DDs

- Arachnoid cyst: CSF-density, non-enhancing lesion, most frequently seen in the middle cranial fossa. Absence of any restricted diffusion is the main differentiating feature.
- Other intracranial cystic lesions such as neurenteric cyst, hydatid cyst, dermoid cyst.

MANAGEMENT

Surgical excision.

Central Neurocytoma

This WHO grade II intraventricular tumor, usually attached to the septum pellucidum, arises from subependymal neural progenitor cells. It typically affects young adults (20–40 years) and

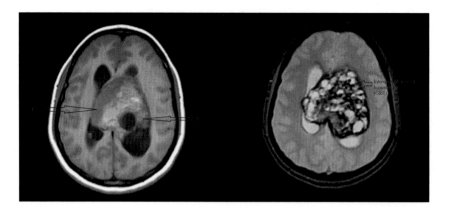

Figure 4.8 Central neurocytoma.

generally has a good prognosis. Most common location is lateral ventricles around foramen of Monro.

CLINICAL

Symptoms of raised intracranial pressure, headaches and seizures (if extraventricular extension is seen).

IMAGING

- NCCT – well-defined, lobulated, usually hyperattenuating lesion with interspersed cystic regions and punctate calcifications, resulting in obstructive hydrocephalus.
- CECT – moderate enhancement.
- MRI – heterogeneous lesion that is iso- to hypointense on T1W and hyperintense on T2W and FLAIR sequences with multiple cystic areas (bubbly appearance), and moderate contrast enhancement. Interspersed hypointense areas are due to calcification or hemorrhage.
- DWI – restricted diffusion of the solid component.
- MRS – elevated choline and glycine peak.

DDs

- Subependymoma – no or minimal enhancement; common in individuals >40 years of age.
- Ependymoma – more typical in the 4th ventricle, and in children. This tumor tends to extend through the foramen.
- SEGA – look for other features of tuberous sclerosis.

- Intraventricular oligodendroglioma – calcifications are large and irregular.
- Intraventricular meningioma – well-circumscribed mass, homogeneous post-contrast enhancement.
- Choroid plexus papillomas – common in children, intense post-contrast enhancement.

MANAGEMENT

Complete surgical resection with adjuvant chemo- and radiotherapy.

Medulloblastoma

Most common malignant brain tumor of childhood, particularly common in males and with a mean age group of more than four years. A rapidly growing, posterior fossa midline mass arises in the region of the cerebellar vermis and the roof of the 4th ventricle. It is an example of small round blue cell tumors.

CLINICAL

Features of cerebellar dysfunction and elevated ICP.

IMAGING

- NCCT – hyperdense lesion with areas of necrosis, cyst formation, and occasional calcifications in the roof of the 4th ventricle with features of obstructive hydrocephalus and surrounding vasogenic edema.
- CECT – moderate to intense heterogeneous enhancement.
- MRI – heterogeneously hypointense on T1W and hyperintense on T2W and FLAIR

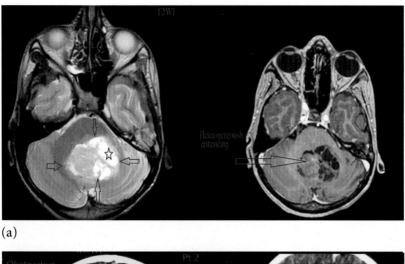

(a)

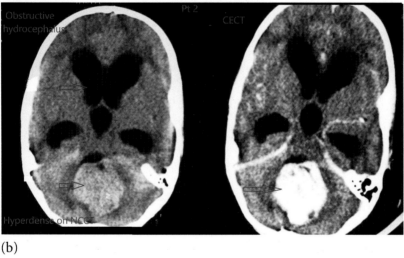

(b)

Figure 4.9 (a) MRI findings of medulloblastoma, (b) CT findings of medulloblastoma.

sequences, with surrounding edema and moderate contrast enhancement. CSF seeding is frequent, warranting the need for imaging of the whole neuraxis to diagnose drop metastasis and leptomeningeal spread.

- DWI – high signal.
- MRS – high choline peak and reduced NAA.

DDs

- Ependymoma – arises from the floor of the 4th ventricle, not showing much DWI restriction, expands the 4th ventricle, and also seen entering into the foramen of Luschka and Magendie.
- Atypical teratorhabdoid tumor (ATRT) – highly aggressive, bulky, heterogeneous mass with calcifications, eccentric cysts,

off-midline location in posterior fossa; common in children younger than three years.

- Pilocytic astrocytoma.
- Exophytic brainstem glioma.

MANAGEMENT

- Radiosensitive tumor
- Surgical resection, radiation therapy, and chemotherapy

Pineoblastoma

An aggressive, round blue cell tumor located in the pineal region. When it is associated with

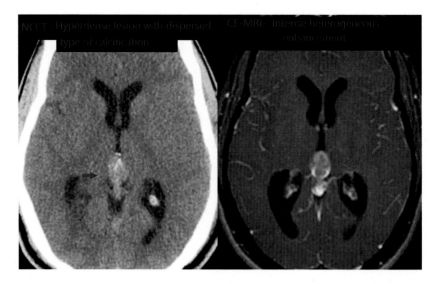

Figure 4.10 Imaging findings of pineoblastoma.

hereditary retinoblastoma, it is called a trilateral retinoblastoma.

CLINICAL

Obstructive hydrocephalus (compression of the cerebral aqueduct) and Parinaud syndrome (compression of the tectal plate).

IMAGING

- CT – ill-defined, lobulated, hyperdense (due to high cellularity) lesion with intense, heterogeneous contrast enhancement due to interspersed areas of hemorrhage and cysts
- Exploded/dispersed type of calcification is characteristic
- Frequent CSF seeding and invasion of adjacent brain structures necessitates the screening of the whole neuraxis
- MRI – T1 and T2 isointense lesion with intense, heterogeneous contrast enhancement and restricted diffusion of the solid component

DDs

- Pineocytoma mature, well-differentiated, low-grade, slow-growing, T2-hyperintense, benign tumor of adults with infrequent CSF seeding
- Germinoma – homogeneous tumor with rare cystic components and intense contrast enhancement, marked male predominance, and characteristic engulfed pattern of calcification

- Teratomas – interspersed lipid-dense areas with elevated alpha-fetoprotein (AFP) and human chorionic gonadotrophin (HCG)

MANAGEMENT

Combination of surgery, chemotherapy, and radiation, with poor prognosis.

ANCILLARY

The pineal gland, a small, conical structure in the quadrigeminal cistern posterior to the 3rd ventricle, can have physiological calcifications, but calcifications with a diameter greater than 1 cm or before the age of 10 are mainly pathological.

Choroid Plexus Papilloma

Benign, slow-growing tumor, most common in male infants, with the most common site being the atrium of the lateral ventricle in children, and the 4th ventricle in adults.

CLINICAL

Symptoms of raised ICP and overproduction hydrocephalus.

IMAGING

- CT scan – lobulated, cauliflower-shaped, iso- to mildly hyperattenuating intraventricular lesion, with punctate calcifications.
- Avid homogeneous enhancement.

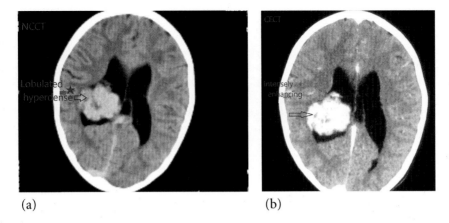

(a) (b)

Figure 4.11 (a and b) CT findings of choroid plexus papilloma.

- MRI – T1 isointense and T2 hyperintense lesion with interspersed signal voids. The lesion shows intense homogeneous enhancement. Spinal cord should be screened to rule out drop metastasis in atypical cases or carcinomas.
- Angiography – intense vascular blush and enlarged feeding choroidal arteries (owing to tumor hypervascularity).

Parenchymal invasion, heterogeneity of the lesion suggests carcinomatous degeneration.

DDs

- Choroid plexus carcinoma can be differentiated predominantly by histologic findings
- Intraventricular meningioma
- Metastasis from bronchogenic carcinoma (in adults)

MANAGEMENT

Surgical resection.

Colloid Cyst

Benign tumor of endodermal origin, usually in young adults.

CLINICAL

Detected incidentally or patients may present with paroxysmal headache, with a change in head position and symptoms of raised intracranial pressure. It may result in coma or sudden death.

IMAGING

- CT – well-defined, round, non-enhancing, homogeneously hyperdense or isodense lesion located anterior to the 3rd ventricle/foramen of Monro, resulting in dilatation of the anterior 3rd ventricle and lateral ventricles, with normal posterior 3rd and 4th ventricle. Mucoid/proteinaceous material in the cyst leads to its hyperdense appearance.
- MRI – T1-hyperintense and T2-hypointense lesion; may show faint rim enhancement.

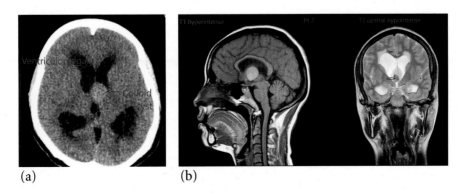

(a) (b)

Figure 4.12 (a) CT of colloid cyst, (b) MRI of colloid cyst.

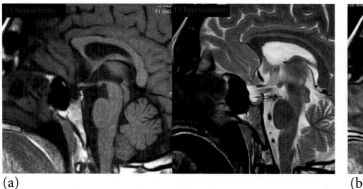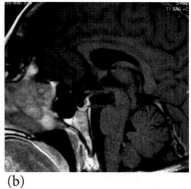

(a) (b)

Figure 4.13 (a and b) MRI findings of Rathke's cleft cyst.

DDs

- Choroid plexus cyst
- Arachnoid cyst of lateral ventricle
- Basilar tip aneurysm mimics colloid cyst on NCCT scan
- Calcified/hyperdense meningioma
- Subependymal giant cell astrocytoma

MANAGEMENT

Symptomatic lesions are treated by shunting or endoscopic surgical resection.

Rathke's Cleft Cyst

Benign, epithelial cyst, originating from the remnants of the embryological Rathke's pouch; usually particularly common in adult females.

CLINICAL

Asymptomatic/headache, visual field defects (bitemporal hemianopsia), hypopituitarism.

IMAGING

- CT scan – intra/suprasellar hypodense lesion.
- Enhancing rim of compressed pituitary surrounding non-enhancing cyst ("claw" sign). Non-enhancing intracystic nodule is characteristic.
- MRI – CSF intensity on T1 and T2WI but the signal intensity may vary depending on the contents of the cyst.

DDs

- Craniopharyngioma - suprasellar, enhancing, and containing calcifications
- Cystic pituitary adenoma may contain fluid-fluid levels and may extend laterally
- Arachnoid cyst

MANAGEMENT

Surgical resection, if symptomatic.

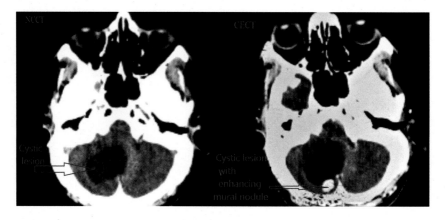

Figure 4.14 CT findings of hemangioblastoma.

Hemangioblastoma

Benign, highly vascular, capillary-rich neoplasm, usually located in the cerebellum in young adult males.

CLINICAL

Headache, cerebellar dysfunction, and altered mental status.

IMAGING

- CT – cystic lesion with isodense mural nodule.
- CECT – intense enhancement of the mural nodule. No cyst wall enhancement is noted.
- MRI – intra-axial, cystic CSF intensity lesion with enhancing pial-based mural nodule and serpentine flow voids. It may result in the displacement of the effaced 4th ventricle.
- Angiography – dilated feeding arteries and draining veins with a dense tumor blush.

DDs

- Juvenile pilocytic astrocytoma – in 5–15 years-of-age group, presents as a laterally located cyst with a well-defined solid component. Cyst wall enhancement may be seen.
- Metastasis from breast, lung –– in elderly patients.
- Pleomorphic xanthoastrocytoma – supratentorial (temporal lobe).
- Ganglioglioma – cortical-based lesion with calcifications; common in the temporal lobe.

MANAGEMENT

Surgical resection with adjuvant radiotherapy.

ANCILLARY

Cerebellar hemangioblastomas have a high rate of recurrence and can involve multiple sites –spinal cord, retina, liver, and pancreas. Hence, ophthalmological examination, annual abdominal sonography, brain/spine MRI screening, and follow-up are all recommended.

Primary CNS Lymphoma (PCNSL)

Rare, highly aggressive B-cell non-Hodgkin lymphoma that involves the brain, spine, cerebrospinal fluid (CSF), and eyes. The lesions are frequently located in the basal ganglia or periventricular white matter and corpus callosum.

CLINICAL

Symptoms of increased ICP, seizures, cognitive decline, and focal neurological deficits.

IMAGING

- CT – hyperdense lesion (due to high cellularity).
- CECT – strong homogeneous enhancement. Ring enhancement is more commonly seen in immunocompromised patients.
- MRI – T1-isointense to hypointense and T2- iso- to hyperintense lesion with strong homogeneous enhancement. Subependymal extension and midline crossing of the corpus callosum may occur.
- DWI – restricted diffusion.
- PWI – low regional cerebral blood volume (rCBV) or only moderate increase in rCBV which is lower than other tumors with extensive neovascularization like GBMs and metastasis.
- Increased uptake on ^{18}F-FDG and ^{11}C-methionine PET scan.
- MRS – glutamate and glycine peak apart from reduced NAA and elevated choline.

DDs

- High-grade gliomas – heterogeneous enhancement, no restricted diffusion.
- Secondary CNS lymphoma – common in immunocompromised patients and tends to involve leptomeninges.
- Tumefactive demyelinating lesions are usually T2-hyperintense and have low rCBV.
- Metastases – multiple, have disproportionate edema and high rCBV.
- Toxoplasmosis encephalopathy presents with fever and commonly involves basal ganglia and gray–white matter junction. The lesions are multifocal, T2-hyperintense with moderate vasogenic edema, lack of subependymal extension, and do not exhibit high uptake on PET scan. MRS shows a lipid-lactate peak.
- Brain abscess – thick, irregular rim of peripheral enhancement, and central restriction of diffusion.

MANAGEMENT

Steroids shrink the tumor effectively. Radiotherapy and chemotherapy with high-dose methotrexate,

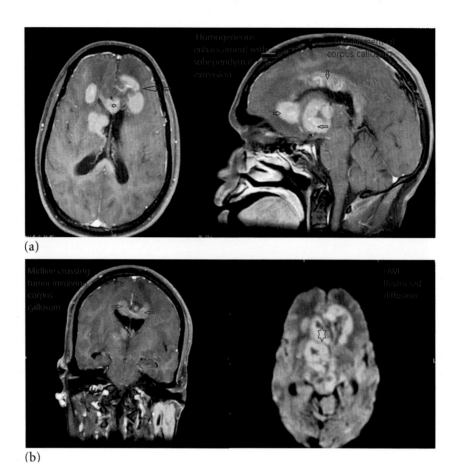

Figure 4.15 (a and b) MRI findings of CNS lymphoma.

cyclophosphamide, hydroxydaunomycin (doxorubicin), vincristine, cytosine arabinoside.

ANCILLARY

- PCNSL is a radio-sensitive and chemo-sensitive tumor.
- Lymphomatosis cerebri, a rare variant of PCNSL, has a bilateral, diffuse, infiltrative appearance rather than a discrete mass. It involves both the deep gray matter nuclei and the white matter tracts, shows hyperintense signal on T2WI and no or patchy contrast enhancement.
- In immunocompromised patients, CNS lymphomas may appear cavitary and difficult to differentiate from other opportunistic infections.

Brainstem Glioma

It is among the most common solid tumors in children, with poor prognosis, and the pons is the most frequent location.

CLINICAL

Cranial nerve deficits, ataxia, long-tract signs, and obstructive hydrocephalus due to compression of the fourth ventricle.

IMAGING

- CT – non-enhancing, hypodense lesion, causing expansion of the pons.
- MRI – expansile, infiltrative T1-iso-/hypointense, T2-hyperintense lesion with no/mild enhancement that tends to encase the basilar artery and flattens the anterior end of the 4th ventricle. No restricted diffusion is noted.

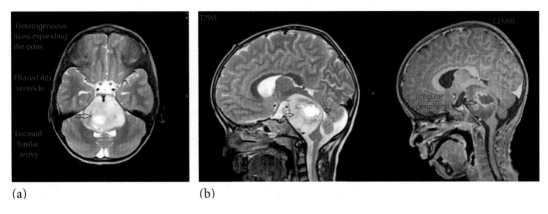

Figure 4.16 (a and b) MRI findings of pontine glioma.

DDs

- Lymphoma
- Granulomatous disease
- Osmotic demyelination
- Disseminated encephalomyelitis

MANAGEMENT

Not suitable for surgery owing to its location in the brainstem and its infiltrative nature. Radiotherapy is the treatment of choice.

ANCILLARY

Focal, dorsal, exophytic, and cervicomedullary gliomas are WHO grade I and II tumors with good prognoses, and are amenable to surgical resection.

Dorsal intrinsic pontine gliomas (DIPG) are WHO grade III tumors with poor prognosis.

Brainstem gliomas are infrequent in adults.

Dysembryoplastic Neuroepithelial Tumors (DNET)

Benign, slow-growing glial-neuronal tumors, common in children and young adults, particularly in the temporal lobes and associated with adjacent cortical dysplasia.

CLINICAL

Intractable partial seizures.

IMAGING

- CT – well-circumscribed, non-enhancing, cortical-based hypodense lesion without any mass effect or peritumoral edema. It may result in remodeling of the inner table of calvarium. Calcifications +/−.
- MRI –T1-hypointense, T2-hyperintense lesion with characteristic 'soap bubble" appearance,

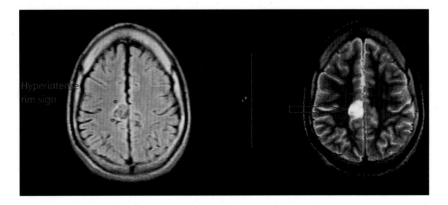

Figure 4.17 Imaging findings of DNET.

minimal edema and mild heterogeneous enhancement.

- FLAIR – "hyperintense rim" sign – hypointense lesion with a thin rim of well-defined hyperintensity at the borders of the DNET, separating it from the surrounding normal brain.

DDs

- Ganglioglioma – cortical, heterogeneously enhancing tumor without any bubbly appearance
- Multi-vacuolating neuronal tumor (MVNT) –bubbly appearance but located in the juxtacortical white matter and does not suppress on FLAIR

- Pleomorphic xanthoastrocytoma (PXA) – cystic tumor with a strongly enhancing mural nodule, often with an adjacent dural tail of enhancement

MANAGEMENT

Surgical resection.

Primitive Neuroectodermal Tumor (PNET)

Better known as embryonal tumor with multilayered rosettes (ETMR) in the recent WHO classification, it is among the most aggressive tumors, with poor prognosis in children.

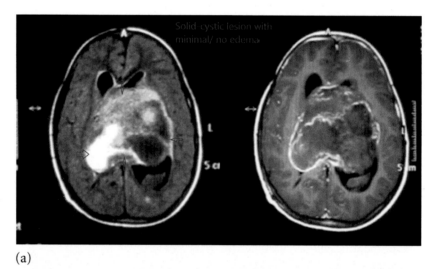

(a)

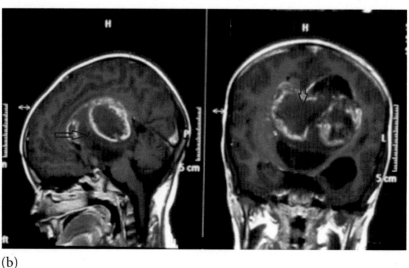

(b)

Figure 4.18 (a and b) MRI findings of PNET.

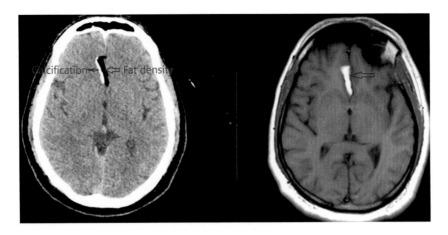

Figure 4.19 Imaging findings of intracranial lipoma.

CLINICAL

Symptoms of raised ICP and focal neurological deficits.

IMAGING

- CT – iso- to hyperdense (owing to high cellularity), large, irregular solid-cystic lesions, with frequent calcifications, absent/minimal peritumoral edema, and heterogeneous contrast enhancement
- MRI – T1 hypo- to isointense, T2 heterogeneous and FLAIR isointense lesion with non-homogeneous enhancement
- Leptomeningeal/subarachnoid seeding is frequent, warranting the imaging of the whole neuraxis
- DWI – restricted diffusion
- MRS – elevated choline, reduced NAA, and specific taurine peak

DDs

- Astrocytoma
- ATRT (Atypical teratorhabdoid tumor)
- Medulloblastoma
- Ependymoblastoma

MANAGEMENT

Surgical resection.

Intracranial Lipoma

Non-neoplastic, congenital lesions commonly located at pericallosal region, quadrigeminal cistern.

CLINICAL

Asymptomatic/seizures, headache.

IMAGING

- CT – non-enhancing, fat density (negative attenuation)
  - May be associated with peripheral calcification
- MRI – hyperintense on T1W and T2WI and becomes suppressed on fat-saturation sequences

DDs

- Intracranial dermoid
- Teratoma

Ruptured Intracranial Dermoid Cyst

Rare lesion with sebum, hair follicles, sweat glands, and more frequently affects females.

CLINICAL

Headache, seizures, vasospasm.

IMAGING

CT:

- Well-defined, lobulated, non-enhancing, low-attenuation (fat density with negative HU), with similar density droplets in subarachnoid spaces and ventricles
- Peripheral rim of calcification +/–

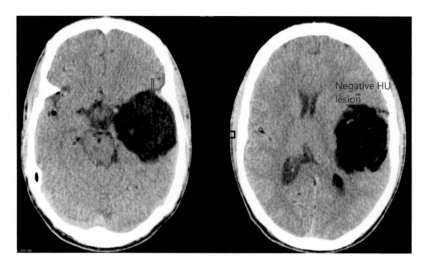

Figure 4.20 CT findings of ruptured intracranial dermoid cyst.

MRI:

- T1-hyperintense, T2 variable signal intensity

DDs

- Intracranial lipoma
- Teratoma
- Epidermoid – restricted diffusion

CNS Metastasis

Multiple/solitary, occur at gray–white matter junction, and primary tumors including breast, lung, renal, melanoma, etc.

CLINICAL

Headaches, seizures, vomiting, altered mental status.

IMAGING

- CT – hypo-/iso-/hyperdense lesions with disproportionate edema
- CECT – strong, nodular, or ring enhancement
- MRI – TI-hypointense (hyperintense, if hemorrhagic), T2/FLAIR hyperintense with variable enhancement pattern
- MRS – elevated choline and reduced NAA
  - Lipid peak (necrosis)
- MR perfusion – elevated rCBV
- ADC – high signal (facilitated diffusion)

DDs

- Primary neoplasm
- Abscess
- Subacute infarct

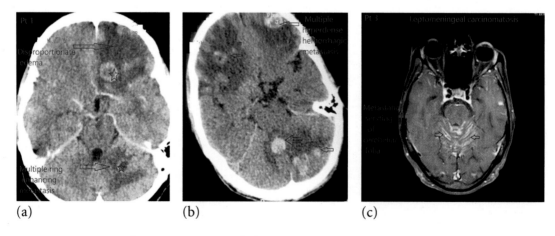

(a)   (b)   (c)

Figure 4.21 (a) Ring-enhancing metastasis, (b) hyperdense hemorrhagic metastasis, (c) leptomeningeal carcinomatosis.

MANAGEMENT

Symptomatic, palliative treatment.

ANCILLARY

- Pachymeningeal – dural based-hyperdense and focal nodular/diffusely enhancing (DD- meningioma)
- Leptomeningeal carcinomatosis – metastatic seeding of subarachnoid space, predominantly basilar cisterns and cerebellar folia with meningitis as a differential diagnosis
- Calcified metastases – osteosarcoma, adeno-carcinoma, lung
- Cystic metastases – papillary cystadenocarcinoma
- Hemorrhagic metastases – melanoma, renal cell carcinoma, thyroid cancer, choriocarcinoma
- Calvarial metastases – lytic in nature

SUGGESTED READING

Adam, A. *Grainger & Allison's Diagnostic Radiology: A Textbook of Medical Imaging.* Churchill Livingstone; 2008.

Johnson, DR, Guerin, JB, Giannini, C, Morris, JM, Eckel, LJ, Kaufmann, TJ. 2016. Updates to the WHO brain tumor classification system: What the radiologist needs to know. *Radiographics* 2017;37(7):2164.

Osborn, AG, Salzman, KL, Jhaveri, MD, Barkovich, AJ. *Diagnostic Imaging: Brain.* Elsevier Health Sciences; 2015.

Watson, N, Watson, NA. *Jones H. Chapman & Nakielny's Guide to Radiological Procedures.* Elsevier; 2018.

5

Infections and Inflammatory Diseases

CONGENITAL BRAIN INFECTIONS

Group of viral, bacterial, and protozoan infections that gain access to the fetal bloodstream transplacentally, resulting in severe fetal anomalies or even fetal loss.

TORCH complex:
T – Toxoplasmosis
O – Other infections (varicella-zoster, parvovirus B19, hepatitis B)
R – Rubella
C – Cytomegalovirus
H – Herpes simplex virus-2

CLINICAL

Developmental delay, failure to thrive.

IMAGING AND DDs

See Table 5.1.

Other differentials include congenital Zika virus, which is an intensely neurotropic virus and presents with microcephaly, ventriculomegaly, calcifications at gray–white matter junction, premature closure of anterior fontanelle, callosal dysgenesis, and neuronal migration abnormalities.

Acute Pyogenic Meningitis

Infection of the meningeal coverings of the brain can be pyogenic (bacterial), acute lymphocytic (viral), or chronic (TB, granulomatous).

- Routes of spread:
  - Hematogenous seeding: Blood–brain and blood–CSF barriers must be breached
  - Direct spread from sinuses/mastoid/fractures
- Common causative organisms vary with age, demography, and immune status

CLINICAL

Neck stiffness, fever, headache, altered sensorium
Gold standard of diagnosis: CSF culture and microscopy

IMAGING

- NCCT – Normal or hydrocephalus with blurred ventricular margins
- CECT – Enhancing exudates extending into sulci
- MRI
  - T1/T2 – Isointense exudates, dirty CSF
  - FLAIR – No suppression, hyperintense sulcal spaces, and CSF
  - CEMRI – Enhancement of pial surfaces
  - Post-contrast T2–FLAIR images and delayed T1 post-contrast images help in identification of subtle cases
  - DWI – Restriction seen in subarachnoid spaces

ORGANISM–SPECIFIC IMAGING FEATURES

- Citrobacter – rapidly cavitating white matter lesions
- Fungal – thick and nodular meningeal enhancement
- Tuberculosis – basal exudates and thick meningeal enhancement

COMPLICATIONS

- Extraventricular obstructive hydrocephalus
- Choroid plexitis and ventriculitis
- Cerebritis, brain abscess

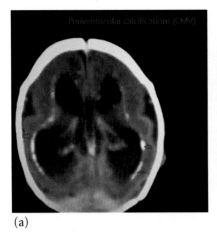 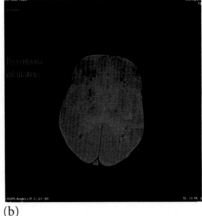

| (a) | (b) |

Figure 5.1 (a) Periventricular calcifications of CMV, (b) periventricular calcifications on MRI.

Table 5.1 Imaging Findings of CMV and Its Differentials

	CMV	Toxoplasmosis	HSV	HIV	Rubella
CT	Periventricular calcifications	Cortical and subcortical calcifications	Hemorrhagic foci in cortex and basal ganglia calcifications absent	Basal ganglia calcification	Parenchymal calcifications
MRI	Microcephaly Ventriculomegaly Periventricular cysts Migration abnormalities Volume loss	Ventriculomegaly Multiple subcortical cysts	Cortical and subcortical white matter band – hypointense on T1W and hyperintense on T2W	Frontal lobe atrophy Ectasia of intracranial arteries	Multiple foci of T2/FLAIR hyperintensities

- Empyemas, subdural effusions
- Vasculitis, thrombosis, infarcts

DDs

Imaging features of acute pyogenic meningitis are very non-specific and can be seen under a variety of conditions. Clinical correlation plays an important role.

- Subarachnoid hemorrhage:
  - Hyperintense on T1
  - History of trauma/presence of any intraparenchymal bleed
- Neurosarcoid – pituitary involvement
- Meningeal metastases/leptomeningeal carcinomatosis with known primary (breast, lung)
- Chemical meningitis in cases of ruptured dermoid with no history of fever

MANAGEMENT

Antibiotic therapy.

Subdural Empyema with Cerebral Abscess

Crescentic, extra-axial collection of purulent material between the cranial dura and the arachnoid mater that does not cross the midline; usually associated with sinusitis and mastoiditis.

CLINICAL

Fever, vomiting, neurological deficits, impaired consciousness.

IMAGING

- CT – hypodense collection with rim enhancement

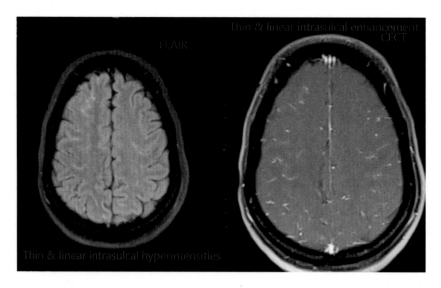

Figure 5.2 MRI findings of meningitis.

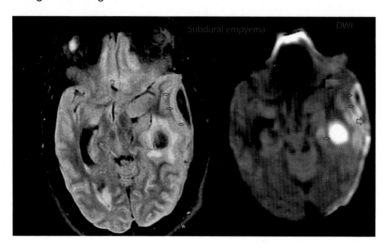

Figure 5.3 MRI findings of subdural empyema with cerebral abscess.

- • Adjacent mass effect
- • Look for associated venous thrombosis, abscess, infarction
- MRI – lesion is isointense on T1W (owing to proteinaceous contents), hyperintense on T2WI with rim enhancement
- DWI – shows restriction

DDs

- Subdural sterile effusions – hypointense on T1WI, without any restricted diffusion
- Chronic subdural hematoma – hyperintense on T1WI
- Epidural abscess – biconvex shape, can cross the midline, and adjacent brain parenchyma usually appears normal

MANAGEMENT

- Antimicrobial therapy
- Surgical drainage

Otogenic Brain Abscess

CLINICAL

Seizures, headache, projectile vomiting, otorrhea.

IMAGING

- CT – opacified mastoid air with the erosion of the cortex and sigmoid plate
  - Ring-enhancing hypodense lesion with adjacent edema

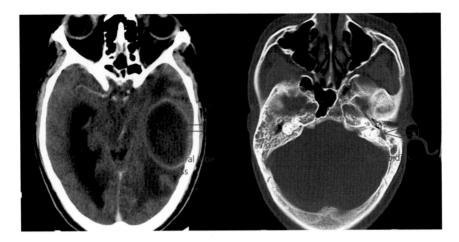

Figure 5.4 Brain abscess due to mastoiditis.

- MRI – lesion is heterogeneously hypointense on T1W, hyperintense on T2WI with ring enhancement

Look for associated signs of sinus thrombosis.

MANAGEMENT

Surgical exploration with symptomatic treatment.

ANCILLARY

Avoid lumbar puncture to prevent coning.

Temporal abscess occurs via erosion of tegmen tympani, and cerebellar abscess occurs *via* Trautmann's triangle.

Cerebral Abscess

Localized infection of brain parenchyma, which can affect any age group with uncorrected cyanotic heart diseases, trauma, endocarditis, sinonasal/orbital/dental/mastoid infections as predisposing factors.

IMAGING AND DDs

Cerebral abscess evolves in four stages. Imaging features and differentials vary accordingly.

- GRE – blooming may be seen
- MRS – amino acids, lactate, acetate peaks in the necrotic core
- Perfusion study – abscess wall (fibrotic capsule) – low rCBV

Neurocysticercosis (NCC)

This is the most common parasitic infection of CNS, caused by *Taenia solium* (pork tapeworm) *via* the fecal-oral route.

CLINICAL

Headache, seizures.

IMAGING

The disease process occurs in four stages.

Usually, multiple lesions, in different stages of development, can be seen, which is characteristic of NCC (see Table 5.3).

Scolex (the anterior segment of the tapeworm) is hyperintense to CSF, non-enhancing, and may show restriction.

LOCATIONS

- Parenchymal > subarachnoid > intraventricular > spinal
- *Subarachnoid NCC* are extra-axial lesions but can cause overlying fibrosis, become "sealed" in the CSF cleft, and appear intra-axial:
  - Racemose NCC
  - "Grape-like" lesions in subarachnoid space, most commonly basal cisterns
  - No identifiable scolex
  - Are multiple variable-sized bunches of cysts
  - Show rim enhancement
  - Cause complications like obstructive hydrocephalus, vasculitis, and infarcts

Table 5.2 Imaging Findings and DDs of Four Stages of Cerebral Abscess

	Early Encephalitis	Late Encephalitis	Early Encapsulation	Late Encapsulation
Time	Days 1–2	Days 2–7	1–2 weeks	2 weeks – a few months
Key features	Focal area of inflammation with no visible necrosis	Central necrosis develops Incomplete abscess wall	Complete well-defined abscess wall develops	Abscess shrinks in size, wall thickens, and edema reduces.
CT	Ill-defined hypodense lesion No enhancement	Irregular incomplete ring enhancement	Well-defined lesion with ring enhancement	May persist as enhancing focus
T1WI	Isointense	Hypointense	Hypointense	Iso-/Hypointense
T2/FLAIR	Hyperintense	Hyperintense	"Double rim" sign (inner hyperintense and outer hypointense rim)	Hyperintense
CEMRI	Patchy enhancement	Irregular, incomplete rim enhancement	Typical ring-enhancing lesion	Shrinking, irregular ring-enhancement
DWI	Faint restriction	Restricts strongly	Necrotic area restricts	Non-specific
DDs	*Stroke* – territorial distribution No history of fever *Low-grade glioma* – no diffusion restriction/ enhancement No history of fever	*Neoplasms* –- high rCBV and choline peak on MRS *Demyelinating disorders* – open ring enhancement and no amino acid peak on MRS	*Ring-enhancing lesions* (Chapter 4)	*Ring-enhancing lesions*

Intraventricular NCC

- Rare, poor prognosis
- Difficult to detect
- Never calcifies
- Best seen on MRI in 3-D sequences, like CISS
- Most common location is 4th ventricle > 3rd > lateral ventricles > aqueduct

Spinal

Extremely rare.

DDs

Depends on location and stage.

- *Intraventricular lesions*
  - Choroid plexus cyst
  - Ependymoma
  - Arachnoid cyst
- *Subarachnoid lesions*
  - Pyogenic meningitis
- *Parenchymal*
  - Tuberculomas
  - Metastasis
  - Other infective granulomas, like toxoplasmosis

MANAGEMENT

Oral albendazole ± steroids.

Tuberculoma

The second most common pattern of CNS tuberculosis (TB), after meningitis, which affects all age

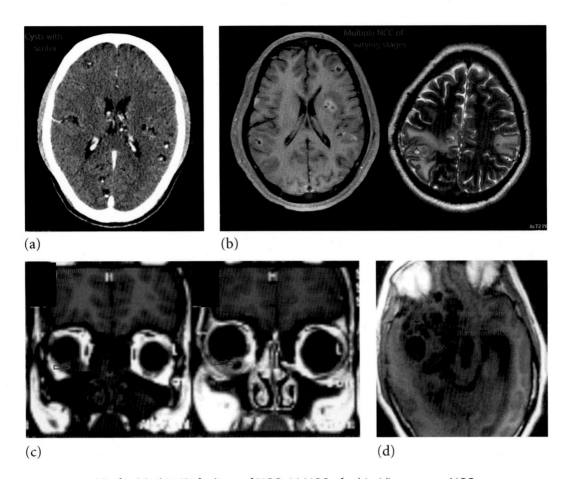

Figure 5.5 (a) CT of NCC, (b) MRI findings of NCC, (c) NCC of orbit, (d) racemose NCC.

Table 5.3 Differentiating Features of Various Stages of NCC

Stage	Vesicular	Colloid Vesicular	Granular Nodular	Nodular Calcified
Disease stage	Viable larva (quiescent/dormant)	Dying	Healed	Healed
Inflammation	Absent	Intense	Reduced	Absent
General imaging features	Cyst with eccentric dot No edema No enhancement	Ring-enhancing lesion with perilesional edema	Faint rim enhancement with reduced edema	Calcified lesions No edema
MRI	Isointense cyst	Mildly hyperintense cystic contents	Thickened, irregular and retracted cyst wall	Calcified nodule (blooming on SWI)
Scolex	T1 hyperintense, non-enhancing	May enhance		

Table 5.4 Differentiating Features between NCC and Tuberculosis

Characteristic	NCC	Tuberculosis
Size	Usually discrete and smaller (< 2 cm)	Usually larger and conglomerated
Location	Gray–white matter junction	Posterior fossa common in midline
Scolex	+	−
Edema	Relatively less	Relatively more
Margins	Smooth	Irregular, shaggy
Other organs commonly involved	Muscles, orbits, skin	Lungs, intestines, lymph nodes
T2WI	Hyperintense	Hypointense
MRS	Amino acid peak	Lipid peak
MT ratio	Higher	Lower
Focal neurological deficits	Less common	More common

groups and presents as a focal brain parenchymal tubercular infection with central caseating necrosis, most commonly caused by *Mycobacterium tuberculosis* (TB) *via* a hematogenous route. They vary in size from 2 cm to giant tuberculomas (4–6 cm). PCR is the best diagnostic modality.

IMAGING

- NCCT – multiple round iso-/hyperdense foci with perilesional edema
- Calcific foci in old head granulomas
- CECT – punctate or ring enhancement
- MRI – lesions are T1 iso-/hypointense, T2 hypointense, and FLAIR hyperintense, with solid or rim enhancement
  - Variable perilesional edema
  - Tuberculomas can rarely present as dural-based enhancing masses
- DWI – solid lesions do not show restriction. Central liquified contents may restrict
- SWI – healed lesions may appear as foci of blooming
- MRS – lipid peak is seen, ↓ NAA/Choline and NAA/Cr ratios
- Perfusion MRI – elevated rCBV in lesion

DDs

- Neurocysticercosis (see Table 5.4)
- Neoplastic lesion (GBM, metastasis)
  - History of known primary
  - GBM is usually larger and crosses the midline
  - Choline is elevated in MRS
- Pyogenic abscess
  - History of predisposing factors
  - Abscess cavity has reduced rCBV
  - Amino acids and lactate peaks on MRS
- Dural-based tuberculoma can mimic meningioma
  - Meningioma is isointense to brain parenchyma
  - Restricts on DWI
  - Different symptomatology

MANAGEMENT

Anti-tubercular therapy.

ANCILLARY

CNS TB can manifest in many forms – meningitis, hydrocephalus, vascular complications, neuropathy, tuberculoma, abscess, miliary TB, focal cerebritis, hypophyseal TB, calvarial osteomyelitis with epidural abscess, and spinal cord tuberculosis (arachnoiditis, spinal cord tuberculoma).

Herpes Encephalitis

Hemorrhagic necrotizing encephalitis is caused most commonly by HSV1 (Herpes simplex virus-1) through reactivation of latent virus from trigeminal nerve ganglia, usually under immunosuppressive conditions. Bilateral but asymmetrical involvement of the limbic system, medial temporal lobe, cingulate, insula, and basifrontal cortex. Brainstem and basal ganglia are usually spared.

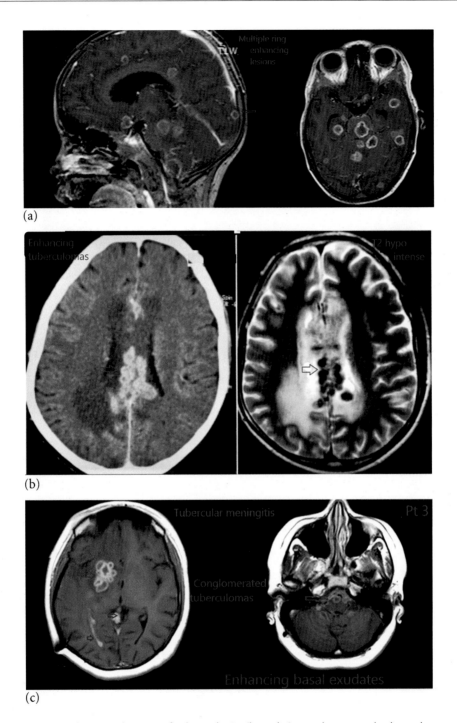

Figure 5.6 (a) Ring-enhancing lesions of tuberculosis, (b and c) conglomerated tuberculomas with basal exudates.

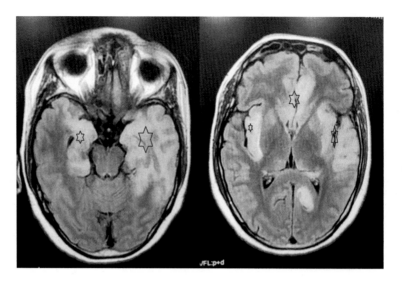

Figure 5.7 Herpetic encephalitis.

In children, HSV2 is the more common causative organism, involving the parietal cortex but sparing the limbic system and the temporal lobes.

CLINICALLY

Fever, seizures, focal neurological deficits, and reduced or altered consciousness.

IMAGING

- CT – hypodensity in involved cortex with effacement of sulci
  - Hemorrhagic areas may present as hyperdensities of CT attenuation >60 HU
- MRI
  - T1 – hypointense with T1 hyperintense hemorrhagic foci

- T2 and FLAIR – hyperintense
- CE-MRI – gyral enhancement
- DWI – restriction present
- SWI – blooming in hemorrhagic areas
- MRS – lactate, choline, myoinositol peaks

DDs

- Limbic encephalitis – paraneoplastic syndrome, associated with carcinoma thyroid. No restricted diffusion and no acute onset.
- Infarct – usually unilateral and involves basal ganglia. Occluded vessels can be seen on an angiogram. No meningeal enhancement.
- Temporal lobe glioma – unilateral, subacute onset. MRS will show choline peak.

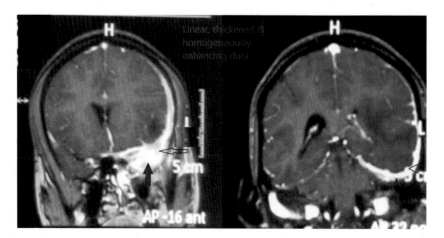

Figure 5.8 Hypertrophic pachymeningitis.

MANAGEMENT

Antiviral and antiepileptic agents.

Idiopathic Hypertrophic Pachymeningitis

Focal fibrotic inflammatory dural thickening usually involves tentorium and falx.

CLINICAL

Headache, cranial neuropathies.

IMAGING

Focal dural thickening that is hyperdense on CT, hypointense on T1 and T2WI, and demonstrates homogeneous dural enhancement (linear/nodular).

Associated mastoiditis, sinus involvement, white matter changes may also be noted.

Biopsy is diagnostic.

DDs

- Dural metastases
- En plaque meningioma
- Granulomatous disease (neurosarcoidosis, Wegener's granulomatosis)

MANAGEMENT

Steroids, immunomodulators, surgical exploration.

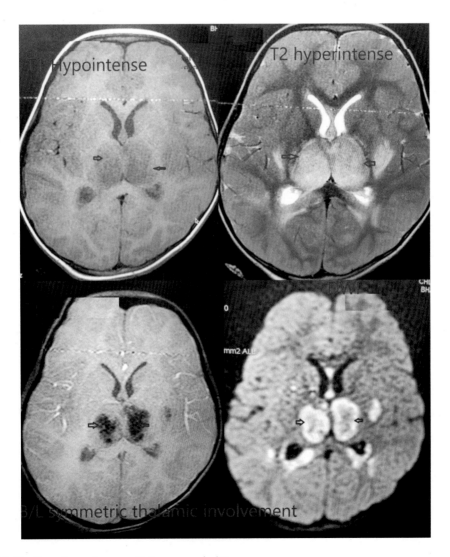

Figure 5.9 Findings in acute necrotizing encephalitis.

Acute Necrotizing Encephalitis

Rare encephalopathy of childhood resulting in multifocal symmetric brain lesions, usually involving the thalamus, putamen, cerebellum, cerebral white matter, internal capsule, and tegmentum.

CLINICAL

History of viral illness followed by sudden-onset neurological deficit.

IMAGING

- CT – bilateral, symmetric hypodense areas usually involving thalamus. Cavitation may occur.
- MRI – T1 hypointense, T2 hyperintense.
- DWI – may reveal diffusion restriction on subacute hemorrhage.
- SWI – if present, petechial hemorrhages are better delineated.

DDs

- Acute disseminated encephalomyelitis – asymmetric involvement and good response to steroids
- Reye syndrome – diffuse cerebral edema, hyperammonemia, lactic acidosis
- Toxic encephalopathies
- Severe hypoxia

MANAGEMENT

Symptomatic and supportive.

SUGGESTED READING

Adam, A. *Grainger & Allison's Diagnostic Radiology: A Textbook of Medical Imaging.* Churchill Livingstone; 2008.

Foerster, BR, Thurnher, MM, Malani, PN, Petrou, M, Carets-Zumelzu, F, Sundgren, PC. Intracranial infections: Clinical and imaging characteristics. *Acta Radiologica* 2007;48(8):875–893.

Osborn, AG, Salzman, KL, Jhaveri, MD, Barkovich, AJ. *Diagnostic Imaging: Brain.* Elsevier Health Sciences; 2015.

6

Disorders Affecting White and Gray Matter: Normal Myelination

A fully myelinated brain appears hyperintense on T1, due to increased lipid content (cholesterol and galactocerebroside), and hypointense on T2, due to the hydrophobic properties of myelin membrane/white matter. The unmyelinated parts of the neonatal brain exhibit T1 hypointensity and T2 hyperintensity relative to the cortex. On a CT scan, non-myelinated white matter (WM) is hypodense in comparison to normal WM and gray matter (GM). MRI is a noninvasive modality of choice, with TI and T2WI as complementary adjuncts, to evaluate the maturation of myelin.

Myelin maturation is a continuous and predictable progressive process in which various parts of the brain are in varying stages of myelination, depending on the age of the infant. Myelination is completed by up to two years of age, correlating concurrently with developmental milestones, though some association tracts, especially around the ventricular trigone, may myelinate after 20–30 years. Axiomatically, maturation progresses from:

- Bottom to top (caudal to rostral)
- Central to peripheral
- Back to front (dorsal to ventral/posterior to anterior)
- Sensory > motor
- Proximal to distal (e.g., optic tracts followed by optic radiations)

As a rule: Brainstem > cerebellum and basal ganglia > cerebral hemisphere (occipital lobe > frontal lobe, and central corona radiata > peripheral white matter of the lobes).

Some exceptions to the rule include frontal (anteriorly) before temporal, and perirolandic

cortex (rostral) before the caudally located anterior limb of the internal capsule.

Multiple factors, like hypoxia, ischemia, infections, congenital, chromosomal, and metabolic abnormalities, hinder the progress of myelination. Hence, it is pivotal to recognize the normal progression of myelin maturation for diagnosing various dysmyelination diseases (leukodystrophies) and demyelinating diseases. The consistent pattern of delayed myelination in two sequential MRI scans, at a minimum gap of six months, indicates hypomyelination.

T1WI is more useful during the first year of life, and minimal change is seen after that. On T2WI, the changes are developing and more prolonged, and hence subtle variations and delays in myelination in the second year are better exhibited. FLAIR follows a pattern similar to that of T2, but which it lags behind. PD-weighted images help in differentiating gliosis from hypomyelination. DWI is highly sensitive in the acute settings. Diffusion tensor imaging (DTI) for measurement of FA (which increases with brain maturation) may also be used for assessment of myelination. Brain maturation is characterized (using MR spectroscopy) as an increase in NAA and creatine and a concomitant decrease in choline, myo-inositol, and lipids.

A normal developmental variant, *Terminal zones of incompletely myelinated brain,* is seen as bilateral, symmetrical foci of high signal in the WM dorsolateral to the atria of the lateral ventricles. It needs to be differentiated from PVL (periventricular leukomalacia). Small bands of low signal (representing normally myelinated brain), separating the high-signal regions from the ventricles, represent

Table 6.1 Myelination Calendar with Red Depicting T1 WI and Blue Delineating T2 WI

Birth	1 Month	2 Months	3 Months	4 Months
Medulla	MCeP	PLIC	Deep cerebellar WM	Splenium
Dorsal pons	ON, OT,	Perirolandic CSO	ALIC	OR
Midbrain	OR	OT	Ventral pons	
PLIC			MCeP	
SICeP				
Perirolandic cortex				
Ventral lateral thalami				
	5 Months	6 Months	7 Months Subcortical	8 Months
		Genu	U-fibers of the	Genu
		Splenium	occipital lobe	ALIC
		Ventral pons		
	9 Months	10 Months	11 Months	12 Months
				Subcortical U-fibers of frontal and temporal lobes
				Deep cerebellar WM
	13 Months	14 Months	15 Months	16 Months
		Frontal WM	Subcortical U-fibers of the occipital lobe	Temporal WM
			Entire posterior fossa	
	17 Months	18 Months	19 Months	20 Months
	21 Months	22 Months	23 Months	24 Months
				Subcortical U-fibers of the frontal and temporal lobes

PLIC – posterior limb of internal capsule
ALIC – anterior limb of internal capsule
MCeP – middle cerebellar peduncle
SICeP – superior and inferior cerebellar peduncles
WM – white matter
ON – optic nerve
OT – optic tract
OR – optic radiation
CSO – centrum semiovale

terminal zones of myelination, but, in PVL, the high signal intensity will extend all the way to the ventricular ependyma.

CLASSIFICATION

WM diseases can be classified as:

1) Demyelinating disorders – secondary destruction of previously myelinated structures. Lesions are generally asymmetrical and multifocal.

2) Dysmyelinating disorders – primary abnormalities of myelin formation, usually resulting from inherited enzyme deficiencies ("inborn errors of metabolism," leukodystrophies). Lesions are generally symmetrical and confluent in nature.

3) Hypomyelination disorders – partial myelination of WM.

Demyelinating Disorders

- Autoimmune – multiple sclerosis and its variants, acute disseminated

encephalomyelitis (ADEM), and acute hemor-rhagic leukoencephalopathy
- Infectious – Lyme disease, progressive mul-tifocal leukoencephalopathy (PML), and human immunodeficiency virus (HIV) encephalopathy
- Vascular – arteriolosclerosis, cerebral amyloid angiopathy (CAA), cerebral autosomal domi-nant arteriopathy with subcortical infarcts and leukoencephalopathy (CADASIL)
- Toxic metabolic processes – methotrexate leukoencephalopathy, and posterior reversible encephalopathy syndrome (PRES)

Dysmyelination Disorders (Leukodystrophies)

Disorders primarily affecting WM, presenting with spasticity, hyperreflexia, and ataxia:

1) Enzyme defect – abnormal formation, destruc-tion or turnover of myelin
2) Single peroxisomal enzyme defect – adrenoleu-kodystrophy (ALD)
3) Lysosomal enzyme disorders – metachromatic leukodystrophy (MLD) and Krabbe disease
4) Cytosolic enzyme defect – Canavan's disease
5) Proteo-lipid protein defect – Pelizaeus-Merzbacher disease
6) Mitochondrial dysfunction – MELAS, Leigh's disease, Kearns-Sayre syndrome

IMAGING
- CT – bilateral hypodense areas; may be sym-metrical. Become more extensive as the disease progresses.
- MRI-T2W – high signal intensity from affected WM.

Metachromatic Leukodystrophy (MLD)

ETIOLOGY
Lack of arylsulfatase-A.

IMAGING
- Moderate ventriculomegaly
- Bilateral, symmetrical demyelination with periventricular and deep WM T2

hyperintensities, with sparing of perivenular WM ("tigroid" pattern)
- Sparing of subcortical U-fibers, especially around atria and frontal horns of the lateral ventricles ("butterfly" pattern)
- NCCT – hypodense lesions, progressing from anterior to posterior in WM
- CECT – no enhancement
- MRI-T2WI – high signal intensity in periven-tricular WM diffusely and cerebellar WM
- Hypointense thalami

Krabbe Disease (Globoid Leukodystrophy)

Symmetrical dysmyelination of the centrum semi-ovale and the corona radiata, and sparing of the subcortical U-fibers.

ETIOLOGY
Lack of P-galactocerebrosidase.

IMAGING
- NCCT – hyperdense basal ganglia, thalami, corona radiata, and cerebellum
- Diffuse hypodensity, involving periventricular WM
- CECT – no enhancement
- MRI – non-specific, confluent symmetrical periventricular WM hyperintensities (WMHs) on T2WI

Alexander Disease

Fibrinoid leukodystrophy, with autosomal reces-sive inheritance.

IMAGING
- NCCT – low attenuation areas in the deep bifrontal WM and basal ganglia
- CECT – mild enhancement in basal ganglia and periventricular region
- MRI – high signal intensity in frontal lobe on T2WI

Canavan's Disease

ETIOLOGY
Deficiency of N-acetyl aspartylase, resulting in accumulation of NAA in urine, plasma, and brain.

Megalencephaly, with involvement of subcortical fibers, along with the globus pallidus, thalamus, and dorsal brainstem, is characteristic.

IMAGING

- NCCT – diffuse hypodensities throughout cerebral WM with normal ventricles
- MRI – homogeneous, symmetrical signal changes throughout the WM bilaterally (low SI on T1W, high SI on T2W)
- MRS – markedly elevated NAA level

Pelizaeus-Merzbacher Disease

ETIOLOGY

Lack of myelin-specific proteolipid apoprotein.

IMAGING

- NCCT – non-specific cerebral and cerebellar atrophy with diffuse hypodensities involving WM
- MRI – diffuse hyperintensities on T2W, interspersed with normal signal intensity in WM, giving "tigroid" pattern due to patchy demyelination
- Thinned-out corpus callosum

Phenylketonuria (PKU)

Disorder involving periventricular WM with sparing of subcortical U-fibers.

ETIOLOGY

Deficiency of phenylalanine hydroxylase, that converts phenylalanine to tyrosine. Its diagnosis is pivotal as timely and appropriate diet restriction can avert neurological deterioration.

IMAGING

- NCCT – periventricular hypodensities
- MRI – hyperintensities involving periventricular deep cerebral WM (mostly optic radiation)

Maple Syrup Urine Disease (MSUD)

ETIOLOGY

Marked generalized edema for 6–7 weeks, then edema decreases. Intense local edema in cerebral peduncles, the posterior limb of the internal capsule, deep cerebellar WM, and the dorsal brainstem.

IMAGING

- NCCT – hypodense globus pallidus and thalamus
- MRI – high signal intensity in globus pallidus and thalamus

Homocystinuria

Mainly affects intracranial vessels, resulting in:

- Multiple small arterial thromboembolic infarcts
- Deep cerebral venous occlusion with infarction
- Superior sagittal sinus thrombosis

Glutaric Aciduria

ETIOLOGY

Type 1 is an autosomal recessive.

- Adversely affects mitochondrial activity
- Deficiency of glutaryl CoA dehydrogenase that converts lysine to tryptophan
- Presentation – progressive dystonia, dyskinesia

IMAGING

- Frontotemporal atrophy
- Batwing dilatation of the Sylvian fissures
- High signal intensity changes in the basal ganglia and caudate nuclei

Methylmalonic Acidemia (MMA)

- NCCT – bilateral hypodensities in the globus pallidus
- MRI – hypointense on T1W and hyperintense on T2W in the globus pallidus

DISORDERS PRIMARILY AFFECTING GRAY MATTER (GM)

GM contains neuronal cell bodies of the CNS.

- Cortical GM of the cerebrum and cerebellum
- Deep GM (nuclei of the basal ganglia, thalami, brainstem, and cerebellum)

Disorders primarily affecting GM present with seizures (cortical GM) and chorea, athetosis, and dystonia (deep GM).

Tay-Sachs Disease

An inherited sphingomyelin lipidosis.

ETIOLOGY

Deficiency of hexosaminidase A.

IMAGING

- CT – symmetric, hyperdense thalami, hydrocephalus, and marked cortical atrophy
- MRI – T2 hyperintense signal in the caudate nuclei, the thalamus, and the putamen

Mucopolysaccharidoses (MPS)

A group of inherited lysosomal storage diseases, characterized by failure to degrade glycosaminoglycans.

MPS 1 (Hurler's Syndrome)

MRI exhibits dilated Virchow-Robin spaces in the peritrigonal areas, dural thickening, and cortical atrophy.

Glycogen Storage Diseases

The patient presents with a varied spectrum of radiographic abnormalities like hepatomegaly, splenomegaly, renomegaly, osseous abnormalities etc.

Mucolipidoses and Fucosidoses

Multisystem involvement with organomegaly and non-specific features.

DISORDERS AFFECTING BOTH GRAY AND WHITE MATTER

Disorders that affect both GM and WM include mitochondrial encephalopathies, Zellweger syndrome, peroxisomal disorders, and multiple sclerosis.

Leigh's Syndrome

A mitochondrial disorder, characterized by subacute necrotizing encephalomyelopathy, with T2-hyperintense, bilateral, symmetrical necrotic lesions in the basal ganglia and brainstem.

Myopathy, Encephalopathy, Lactic Acidosis, and Stroke-Like Episodes (MELAS) Syndrome

Mutation in a mitochondrial gene.

IMAGING

- Multifocal stroke-like cortical lesions (infarcts) crossing the vascular territories, predominantly in the parieto-occipital and parieto-temporal regions
- MRS – elevated lactate levels
- Basal ganglia calcification

BASAL GANGLIA DISORDERS

Includes Hallervorden-Spatz disease, Fahr's disease, Wilson's disease, and Huntington's disease.

PRIMARY NEURODEGENERATIVE CONDITIONS

1) *Dementia*
   - Alzheimer's disease
   - Frontotemporal dementia
   - Lewy body dementia
   - Vascular dementia due to stroke, migraine, CADASIL
2) *Extrapyramidal and other movement disorders*
   - Parkinson's disease, exhibits loss of normal hyperintensity in substantia nigra due to loss of neuromelanin
   - Multisystem atrophy
     - Ponto-cerebellar type with abnormal T2W high signal intensity in the pons in the form of a cross ("hot cross bun" sign)
     - Striatonigral type
   - Huntington's disease – caudate nuclei atrophy
   - Progressive supranuclear palsy – involves the midbrain (tegmentum)
   - Motor neuron disease – involves spinal motor neurons and pyramidal tracts
   - Corticobasal degeneration – asymmetric parietal lobe atrophy
3) *Prion disease*
   - Spongiform encephalopathy – involves GM
   - Creutzfeldt-Jakob disease (CJD) – cortical atrophy with diffuse, symmetrical

hyperintensity on T2WI, and restricted diffusion on DWI in caudate nuclei and the putamen.
- New variant CJD (vCJD) shows symmetrical hyperintensity in the pulvinar of the thalamus
  - Gerstmann-Straussler-Scheinker disease (GSSD) – progressive cerebellar atrophy

4) *Cerebellar atrophy*

Etiology

- Genetic-spinocerebellar atrophy, Friedrich's ataxia (atrophy of the lower brainstem and upper spinal cord), hereditary telangiectasia
- Toxic triggers – phenytoin, alcohol
- Paraneoplastic causes

CASE STUDIES

Multiple Sclerosis

Figure 6.1a and 6.1b illustrate imaging findings of multiple sclerosis.

An autoimmune, inflammatory, demyelinating disease, predominant in young adults and females. It is a chronic relapsing-remitting disease, with a variable clinical spectrum, differing in both space and time (lesions in different regions and of varying ages). Lesions are frequently seen in the periventricular region, the corpus callosum, the callososeptal interface, the brainstem, and the cerebellum.

LABORATORY FINDINGS

- Abnormal (visual evoked potentials [VEPs])
- Immunoglobulin G in serum
- Oligoclonal bands in CSF

IMAGING

- NCCT – iso- to hypodense lesions with associated atrophy of the brain.
- CECT – variable enhancement of active lesions.
- MRI – lesions are iso- to hypointense on T1W (black holes) and hyperintense on T2WI. Acute lesions may show associated edema. T1 hyperintense lesions suggest the progressive nature of the disease.

- FLAIR is better at detection of periventricular plaques.

"Dawson's fingers" refer to initial finger-like thin and linear hyperintensities along the medullary veins, followed by ovoid/elliptical configuration, arranged perpendicularly to the lateral ventricles, extending radially outward and best visualized on sagittal images.

- CE-MRI – incomplete peripheral enhancement around active lesions ("open ring" sign – open component represents the GM side of the lesion, and the enhancing component represents the WM side of the lesion).
- Double inversion recovery (DIR) sequences use two inversion times and better delineate cortical lesions by suppressing both WM and CSF signals.
- Magnetization transfer imaging calculates the ratio (MTR), which is a marker of myelin disorder, a reduction in which favors the diagnosis of multiple sclerosis.
- DTI – increased fractional anisotropy (FA) and diffusivity values.

In a patient with brain lesions, the entire spinal cord and optic nerve should also be scanned.

DDs

- Microvascular ischemic disease – punctate or patchy lesions, frequent in the supratentorial subcortical WM. Spinal cord is usually not affected.
- Acute disseminated encephalomyelitis (ADEM) – monophasic, immune-mediated demyelinating disease with symmetrical, enhancing, diffuse WM abnormalities predominantly involving the cortical and deep GM of the basal ganglia and thalami. It is often seen in children following an infection or vaccination.
- Cerebral autosomal dominant arteriopathy with subcortical infarcts and leukoencephalopathy (CADASIL) – symmetrical, confluent subcortical WM high signal, involving temporal poles and external capsules.
- Progressive multifocal leukoencephalopathy (PML) is caused by reactivation of latent JC polyomavirus in immunosuppressed subjects and is a multifocal demyelinating WM disease.

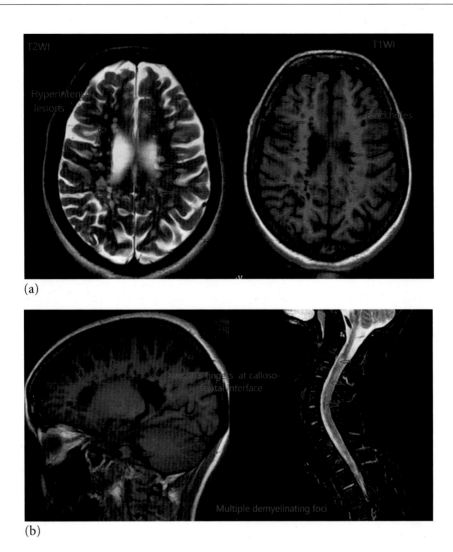

(a)

(b)

Figure 6.1 (a and b) Imaging findings of multiple sclerosis.

It causes confluent WM lesions on MRI, which do not cause mass effect or enhancement. It is relentlessly progressive and usually fatal.

VARIANTS OF MS

- Classic (Charcot type MS).
- Tumefactive MS – it presents as an intraparenchymal lesion with mass effect. Its differentials include abscesses and gliomas, which show closed-ring enhancement.
- Balo's concentric sclerosis – it has alternative bands of demyelination and myelin preservation, usually in a whorl-like manner, and can be visualized as alternating T2-hyperintense and isointense bands.

- Marburg type MS is acute, with fulminating and malignant confluent areas of demyelination, with mass effect and morbidity within a year of onset.
- Schilder type MS is a rare, progressive demyelinating process that begins in childhood. It is characterized by large T2 hyperintense demyelinating plaques in the centrum semiovale region, sparing the cerebral cortex, cerebellum, brainstem, and spinal cord.
- Neuromyelitis optica (NMO) or Devic's disease involves the optic nerves and spinal cord (>3 vertebral segments) along with a few T2 lesions in the brain.

MANAGEMENT

Neuroprotective agents, immunomodulators.

Adrenoleukodystrophy (ALD)

X-linked disease caused by a deficiency of acyl-CoA synthetase.

CLINICAL

Dementia, ataxia, spasticity, cortical blindness, adrenal deficiency.

IMAGING

Bilateral, symmetrical, confluent CT-hypodense and T2-hyperintense areas in the parieto-occipital WM (peritrigonal region) and the splenium of the corpus callosum, sparing the subcortical U-fibers. Dystrophic calcifications in the WM may be seen.

- CECT/MR– enhancement in the advancing rim (serrated rim of contrast enhancement) with a non-enhancing peripheral edematous zone
- MRI – three histopathological zones can be delineated:
  - Central necrotic zone (low SI on T1W and high SI on T2W)

- Middle zone of active demyelination and inflammation (enhances following contrast)
- Peripheral non-enhancing edematous zone (low SI on T1W and high SI on T2W)

DDs

Other leukodystrophies.

MANAGEMENT

Bone marrow transplantation.

Alzheimer's Disease

Most frequently acquired brain degenerative disease with neuronal loss, neurofibrillary tangles, neuritic plaques, and Hirano bodies as predominant microscopic findings.

CLINICAL

Dementia.

IMAGING

- CT – diffusely enlarged ventricles and Sylvian fissures with generalized cortical atrophy and prominent sulci. It has a tendency to spare the cerebellum.
- MRI – reduced cortical GM with disproportionate loss in the anterior temporal lobes (hippocampus), resulting in prominent temporal horns, choroid, and hippocampal fissures. May

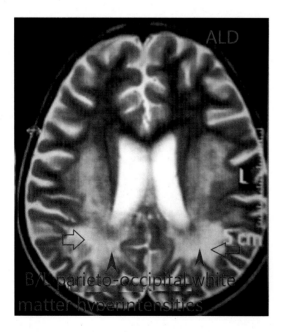

Figure 6.2 Adrenoleukodystrophy.

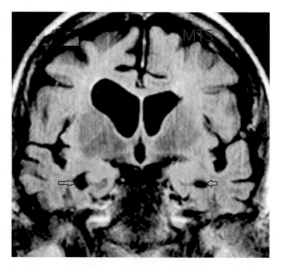

Figure 6.3 Imaging findings of Alzheimer's disease.

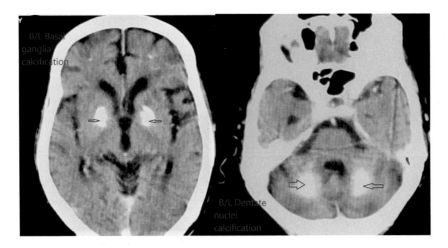

Figure 6.4 Imaging findings of Fahr's disease.

involve medial parietal lobes in later stages. WM hyperintensities (WMHs) are not seen typically.

DDs

- Multi-infarct dementia – severe subcortical and periventricular WM disease
- Normal aging
- Subdural hematoma
- Lewy disease has prominent parkinsonian features with accentuated frontal lobe atrophy
- Pick's disease commonly affects frontal and temporal lobes

Fahr's Disease (Familial Brain Calcification)

Abnormal calcium deposition in the basal ganglia, thalamus, dentate nucleus, cerebellum, subcortical WM, and the hippocampus.

CLINICAL

Neuropsychiatric symptoms without any evidence of specific etiology and abnormality in laboratory findings.

IMAGING

- CT – bilateral, symmetrical basal ganglia calcifications (globus pallidus). It may also involve the caudate nucleus, putamen, thalamus, internal capsule, subcortical, and the cerebellum.
- T1 hyperintense, T2 variable signal intensity.
- GRE (gradient-echo) – hypointense.

DDs

- Idiopathic due to aging (normal)
- Metabolic disorders like hypoparathyroidism, hyperparathyroidism, pseudohypoparathyroidism, and pseudo-pseudohypoparathyroidism
- Postinfectious calcifications (TORCH, neurocysticercosis, tuberculosis, HIV)
- Mitochondrial disorders, like MELAS
- Carbon monoxide and lead intoxication

MANAGEMENT

No specific treatment.

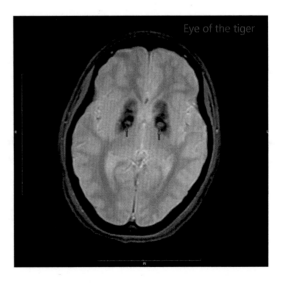

Figure 6.5 "Eye-of-the-tiger" sign.

Hallervordern-Spatz Disease (Pantothenate Kinase-Associated Neurodegeneration, PKAN)

CLINICAL

Progressive dementia, spasticity, dysarthria.

IMAGING

Brain iron accumulation in the globus pallidus, substantia nigra (pars reticularis), and red nuclei, resulting in neurodegeneration.

- CT – bilateral basal ganglia calcification may be seen
- MRI-T2W ("eye of the tiger") – bilateral, symmetrical hypointense signal in the globus pallidus, with central hyperintense spot due to gliosis
- T1W – bilateral hyperintense signal
  - Generalized brain atrophy in later stages
- SWI – susceptibility artifact in the area of iron accumulation
- MRS – reduced NAA peak and elevated myo-inositol peak

MANAGEMENT

Symptomatic treatment.

Non-Ketotic Hyperglycemia-Hemichorea-Hemiballismus (NKHHH Diabetic Striatrophy)

It is associated with non-ketotic diabetic hyperosmolar coma, frequent in elderly females. Usually unilateral, although, unusually, it can also be bilateral infrequently.

CLINICAL

Seizures, vomiting, unilateral involuntary, non-rhythmic movements (chorea and ballismus).

IMAGING

- CT – hyperdense basal ganglia, commonly striatum (the caudate nucleus and putamen), contralateral to the symptomatic side
- MRI – non-enhancing, T1 hyperintense, T2 hypointense signal changes in striatum

DDs

- Wilson's disease – usually involves the thalamus also
- Striatal infarct
- Basal ganglia calcification – bilateral
- Hypertensive hemorrhage
- Carbon monoxide poisoning

MANAGEMENT

Symptoms resolve with correction of glucose levels.

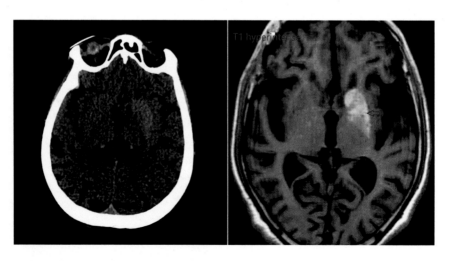

Figure 6.6 Imaging findings of NKHHH.

SUGGESTED READING

Barkovich, AJ. Concepts of myelin and myelination in neuroradiology. *American Journal of Neuroradiology* 2000;21(6):1099–1109.

Cheon, J-E, Kim, I-O, Hwang, YS, Kim, KJ, Wang, K-C, Cho, B-K, Chi, JG, Kim, CJ, Kim, WS, Yeon, KM. Leukodystrophy in children: A pictorial review of MR imaging features. *Radiographics* 2002;22(3):461–476.

Sarbu, N, Shih, RY, Jones, RV, Horkayne-Szakaly, I, Oleaga, L, Smirniotopoulos, JG. White matter diseases with radiologic-pathologic correlation. *Radiographics* 2016;36(5):1426–1447.

Schiffmann, R, van der Knaap, MS. Invited article: An MRI-based approach to the diagnosis of white matter disorders. *Neurology* 2009;72(8): 750–759.

Welker, KM, Patton, A. Assessment of normal myelination with magnetic resonance imaging. *Seminars in Neurology* 2012;32(01):15.

7

CSF Circulation and Disorders

Sources of CSF Production

1) Brain interstitial fluid (ISF) – extra-choroidal source
2) Choroid plexus
3) Ventricular ependyma and brain capillaries – less significant source

In an adult human, the volume of ISF is approximately 280 ml, and that of CSF is about 140 ml (80 ml in the cerebral subarachnoid space (SAS), 30 ml in the ventricles, and 30 ml in the spinal SAS). The SAS lies between the pia and the arachnoid mater. Typically, 500–600 ml CSF are produced daily, at a rate of 0.4 ml/minute.

CSF Drainage

- 1/3 *via* arachnoid granulations in the cranial dura mater
- 1/3 *via* paravascular spaces adjacent to the intracerebral and leptomeningeal arteries to the cervical lymphatics
- 1/3 *via* spinal vessels

CSF Absorption

CSF is absorbed mainly by arachnoid villi into the venous system (mainly the superior sagittal and transverse sinuses).

Ventricles

Ventricles are cavities lined with ependymal cells, formed *via* expansion of the central cavity of the embryonic neural tube.

Lateral Ventricles

- Frontal horns – most anterior segment
- Body/atrium – lies posteriorly under the corpus callosum and contains the choroid plexus
- Occipital horns – lie posteriorly and are lined by white matter (WM) tract (geniculocalcarine tract and forceps major of corpus callosum)
- Temporal horns lie inferiorly
- Foramen of Monro at the junction of the frontal horn and body

3rd ventricle is a slit-like midline cavity between two thalami, and is connected to the 4th ventricle *via* the aqueduct of Sylvius.

4th ventricle is a rhomboid/diamond-shaped cavity between the pons and the cerebellum.

Choroid plexus is highly vascular, with frond-like excrescences covered by ependyma-derived secretory epithelium. It is absent from the cerebral aqueduct, and from the frontal and occipital horns of the lateral ventricles. Not apparent on imaging of the 3rd ventricle.

CSF Flow Pathway

Lateral ventricle → Interventricular foramen of Monro (Y-shaped) → 3rd ventricle
→ Cerebral aqueduct of Sylvius → 4th ventricle
→ Central canal of the spinal cord

Two lateral foramina of Luschka and a medial foramen of Magendie are the natural connections between the ventricular system and the SASs.

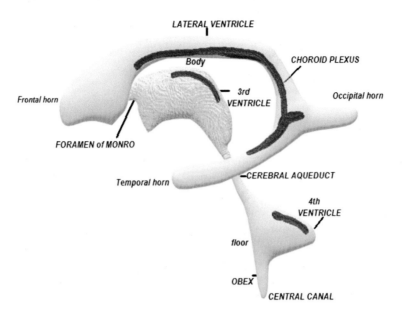

Figure 7.1 CSF flow pathway.

Cisterns

See Figure 7.2.

1) *Suprasellar cistern*
    Five-pointed CSF space, bounded anteriorly by interhemispheric fissures, laterally by Sylvian fissures and posteriorly by the perimesencephalic cistern.
    Contents include:
    • Optic chiasm
    • Pituitary stalk
    • Circle of Willis
    • Internal carotid artery
2) *Perimesencephalic cistern*
    – Interpeduncular cistern anterior to midbrain (upper end of basilar artery, 3rd cranial nerve)
    – Crural cistern lies anterolaterally of the midbrain
    – Ambient cistern lies posterolateral to midbrain (4th cranial nerve)
    – Quadrigeminal plate cistern lies posteriorly (pineal gland and vein of Galen)
3) *Cerebellopontine angle (CPA) cistern*
    – Contains 7th and 8th cranial nerves along with the anterior inferior cerebellar artery (AICA)
4) *Pre-pontine cistern* – contains basilar artery
5) *Pre-medullary cistern* – contains 9th, 10th, and 11th cranial nerves and vertebral artery

6) *Superior cerebellar cistern* – contains vein of Galen
7) *Cisterna magna* is the largest cistern and is also known as the cerebellomedullary cistern.
    • Contents include:
        – Vertebral arteries
        – PICA (posterior inferior cerebellar artery)
        – 9th, 10th, and 11th cranial nerves

CSF Flow Artifacts

CSF flow artifacts on MR scan are due to the pulsatile nature of CSF.

1) Artifacts due to patient's movement; may need verbal reminders and mild sedation
2) Artifacts due to turbulent flow with signal loss in the cerebral aqueduct, 4th ventricle and around the pulsatile vessels (mainly the basilar artery, mimicking aneurysmal dilatation)
3) Artifacts due to time-of-flight (TOF) effects
    • Signal loss (dark CSF), where flow is accelerated through narrow points, like the foramen of Monro
    • Bright CSF, due to incomplete nulling on FLAIR sequence, simulating subarachnoid hemorrhage

Normal Variants

See Figure 7.3.

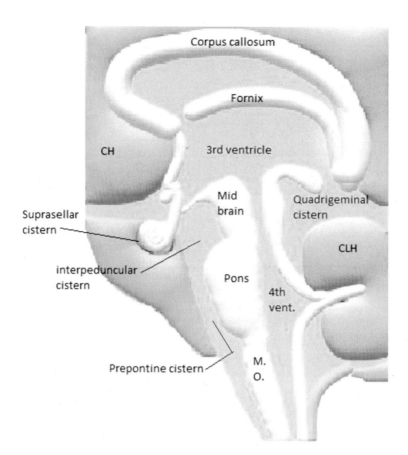

Figure 7.2 Cistern anatomy.

Asymmetric Lateral Ventricles

1) The cavum septum pellucidum (CSP) is a fluid-filled cavity between the frontal horns of the lateral ventricles. The cavum vergae (CV) is the posterior extension of the CSP between the fornices, occurring in conjunction.
2) The cavum velum interpositum (CVI) is a thin triangular CSF space that overlies the thalami and the 3rd ventricle. It typically occurs without CSP, displaces the internal cerebral veins inferiorly, and displays the fornices superiorly.
3) An absent septum pellucidum exhibits a squared-off (box-like) configuration of frontal horns.
4) Mega cisterna magna refers to a retrocerebellar CSF space, measuring more than 10 mm in the mid-sagittal plane.
5) Virchow-Robin spaces, also known as perivascular spaces, are well-defined, CSF density spaces that surround perforating vessels. These are usually found in the basal ganglia region and need to be differentiated from lacunar infarcts. Lacunar infarcts are surrounded by areas of encephalomalacia, best seen as high signal intensity on FLAIR sequences. Giant perivascular (tumefactive) spaces – anterior temporal lobe perivascular spaces are rare, and may mimic a cystic tumor.
6) Arachnoid granulations – arachnoid villus projections into the dural sinuses that allow drainage of CSF from the SAS into the venous system. They are usually located near transverse and superior sagittal sinuses. Well-defined, CSF density, non-enhancing osteolytic lucencies or filling defects in dural venous sinuses. DDs include calvarial metastasis, myeloma lesions, and dural venous thrombosis.

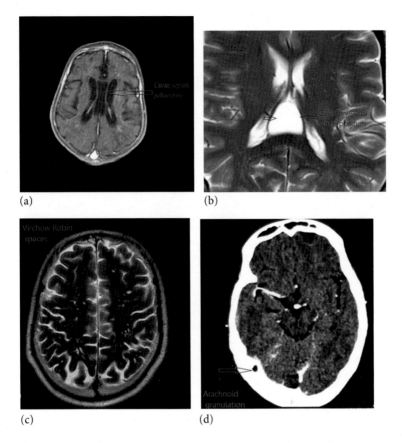

Figure 7.3 (a) Cavum septum pellucidum, (b) cavum vergae, (c) Virchow-Robin spaces, and (d) arachnoid granulation.

CASE STUDIES

Hydrocephalus

Is itself a pathology and a frequent complication of various other pathological ailments; it occurs due to an imbalance between CSF production and absorption, resulting in either overproduction of CSF or a ventricular obstruction causing a CSF accumulation.

CLINICAL

Headache, papilledema, nausea, vomiting, or 6th cranial nerve palsy.

IMAGING

Axial Studies

- Enlarged temporal horn of the lateral ventricle (out of proportion to the basal SAS)
- Rounded appearance of frontal horns
- Lateral ventricular atrial diameter of 10–12 mm (mild), 12–15 mm (moderate) and >15 mm (marked hydrocephalus)
- Effaced cerebral sulci
- Transependymal CSF migration, as the low-density halo in adjacent WM, along with blurring of ventricular margins, is suggestive of acute hydrocephalus
- Parenchymal volume loss

Sagittal

- Thinning and stretching of corpus callosum
- Downward bowing of the 3rd ventricular floor
- Enlarged anterior and posterior recesses

TYPES

See Table 7.1.

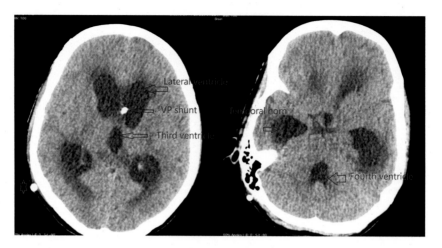

Figure 7.4 Hydrocephalus with VP shunt *in situ*.

Table 7.1 Comparison of Intraventricular and Extraventricular Hydrocephalus

	Intraventricular Hydrocephalus (IVOH)	Extraventricular Hydrocephalus (EVOH)
Type	Non-communicating type	Communicating type
Etiology	• Congenital aqueductal stenosis • Colloid cyst within the foramen of Monro • Obstructing tumor	Usually secondary to hemorrhage or meningitis
Pathology	Occurs due to an obstruction within the ventricular system, resulting in upstream ventricular dilatation	Occurs due to impaired CSF resorption at the arachnoid granulations, without any obstruction within the ventricular system
Management	CSF diversion	Membrane fenestration

DDs

See Table 7.2.

ANCILLARY

Aqueductal stenosis is a frequent cause of congenital and acquired non-communicating hydrocephalus, with congenital causes including aqueductal webs/diaphragms or gliosis, and acquired causes including external compression by tumors or intrinsic abnormalities like infection, inflammation or hemorrhage.

IMAGING

- CT – triventricular (both lateral and 3rd ventricle) hydrocephalus
- MRI
  - Funneling of aqueduct
  - Downward bulging of the 3rd ventricular floor into the interpeduncular cistern
  - Expansion of the suprachiasmatic and suprapineal recesses
  - Normal 4th ventricle
- CSF flow study – absent flow void at the level of the aqueduct

MANAGEMENT

VP shunting or endoscopic third ventriculostomy.

Normal Pressure Hydrocephalus (NPH)

Also known as Adam's syndrome, it is common in the 50–70 age group, with characteristic ventriculomegaly disproportionate to cerebral atrophy and normal CSF pressure.

Table 7.2 Comparison of Hydrocephalus from Cerebral Atrophy

Hydrocephalus	Cerebral Atrophy
All ventricles are enlarged (communicating), 4th ventricle may be normal (non-communicating)	Generalized dilatation (temporal horns normal)
Sulci not enlarged, fissures may be dilated	Sulci enlarged
Disproportionate enlargement of ventricles in comparison to sulci	Proportionate enlargement of ventricles and SASs
Callosal angle <120 degrees	Callosal angle >120 degrees
Interstitial edema present	WM lesions may be seen

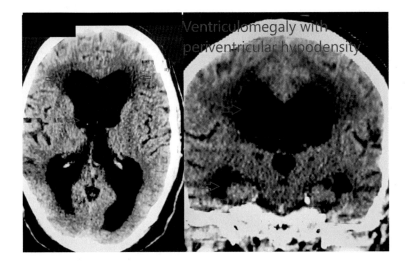

Figure 7.5 CT imaging findings of NPH.

CLINICAL

Triad of:

- Dementia
- Urinary incontinence
- Gait apraxia

IMAGING

- Ventriculomegaly with Sylvian fissure widening
- Periventricular hypodensity on CT and hyperintensity on T2/FLAIR
- PET/SPECT – widespread cortical and subcortical hypometabolism and persistence of radiotracer beyond 24–48 hours in the lateral ventricles
- CSF flow studies – elevated aqueductal CSF stroke volume and peak velocity

- Other causes of ventriculomegaly, like trauma, infection, tumors, subarachnoid hemorrhage, etc., should be ruled out

DDs

- Age-related atrophy
- Alzheimer's disease exhibits characteristic dilatation of parahippocampal fissures

MANAGEMENT

VP shunting for symptomatic relief

Benign Enlargement of Subarachnoid Spaces in Infancy (BESSI)

Self-limiting benign external hydrocephalus due to absorption deficiency in infancy. Normally, seen at 3–8 months, particularly common in males.

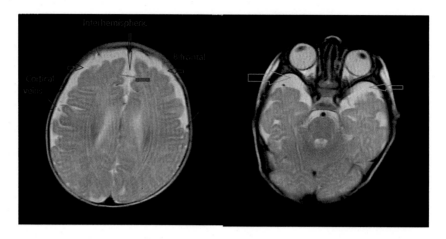

Figure 7.6 MRI findings of BESSI.

CLINICAL

Increasing head circumference (macrocephaly), frontal bossing, widened fontanelle.

IMAGING

- Prominent bifrontal and interhemispheric SAS (>5 mm)
- No significant hydrocephalus
- Cortical vein sign – bridging cortical veins are seen adjacent to inner calvaria, within the SASs, easily seen on Doppler ultrasound, CECT, and MRI (elongated flow voids)

Normal SAS measurements:

- Frontal region – 4 mm
- Anterior interhemispheric fissure – 4 mm
- Sylvian fissure – 3 mm

DDs

- Subdural collection/hemorrhage – look for associated features like retinal hemorrhages, etc., in a child with a history of abuse. Cortical veins are displaced away from the inner table of calvaria, due to compression of SASs by subdural hygromas.
- Type 1 glutaric aciduria – symptomatic infants associated with basal ganglia and WM signal changes.

MANAGEMENT

No treatment required. Self-limiting by 12–24 months.

SUGGESTED READING

Adam, A. *Grainger & Allison's Diagnostic Radiology: A Textbook of Medical Imaging.* Churchill Livingstone; 2008.

Watson, N, Watson, NA, *Jones H. Chapman & Nakielny's Guide to Radiological Procedures.* Elsevier; 2018.

8

Phakomatoses (Neurocutaneous Syndromes)

An assortment of disorders, with variable inheritance patterns and degree of penetrance. Manifestations involving the central nervous system, skin, viscera and connective tissues are noted in all of these. Important ones will be discussed as case studies.

OTHER NEUROCUTANEOUS SYNDROMES

- Rendu-Osler-Weber (ROW) syndrome, Hereditary hemorrhagic telangiectasia (HHT)
  - Cutaneous, mucosal, and visceral telangiectasias
  - Vascular malformations of the brain and spinal cord
  - Pulmonary and hepatic arteriovenous fistula, resulting in infarcts, septic emboli, and abscesses
- Ataxia telangiectasia
  - Telangiectasias on the face and eye (oculocutaneous)
  - Progressive cerebellar atrophy with ataxia
  - Immunodeficiency, resulting in neoplasms, and recurrent eye and sinus infections.
- Cowden syndrome
  - Hamartomatous overgrowth of tissues of embryonic origins
  - Mucocutaneous lesions
  - Tumors of breast, thyroid, colon, and endometrium.
  - If associated with Lhermitte-Duclos disease (LDD, dysplastic cerebellar gangliocytoma), it is known as **CO**wden **L**hermitte **D**uclos syndrome (COLD)

- Wyburn-Mason syndrome
  - Facial and retinal vascular nevi
  - Multiple cerebral arteriovenous malformations, involving the midbrain and the visual pathway
- Klippel-Trenaunay-Weber syndrome (angio-osteo hypertrophy)
  - Cutaneous angiomata
  - Soft tissue or bony hypertrophy
  - Deep parenchymal vascular malformations and angiomas
  - Hemimegalencephaly
- Meningioangiomatosis
  - Hamartomatous meningeal-based lesions with thickened and calcified leptomeninges and blood vessels
- Neurocutaneous melanosis
  - Hairy or deeply pigmented nevi
  - Melanosis of the leptomeninges (intensely enhancing)
- Nevus of Ota syndrome
  - Blue-gray lesions in the dermatomes of the ophthalmic and maxillary divisions of the trigeminal nerve
  - Abnormal meningeal pigmentation
  - Meningeal melanocytomas, melanomas of the choroid and ciliary body, and primary melanomas of the CNS
- Hypomelanosis of Ito
  - Hypopigmented skin lesions
  - Cerebral atrophy, abnormalities of migration, gliosis and white matter (WM) involvement are noted
- Basal cell nevus (Gorlin) syndrome
  - Multiple basal cell carcinomas of the skin

- Skeletal abnormalities, like bifid ribs
- Odontogenic keratocysts of the jaw

CASE STUDIES

Neurofibromatosis Type 1 (NF1, von Recklinghausen Disease)

Autosomal dominant, peripheral type of neuro-fibromatosis (NF), in which cutaneous lesions and tumors usually multiply, both in size and number, with age. Plexiform neurofibromas, the hallmark of NF1, are tortuous serpentine masses along the axis of a major nerve, most commonly involving ophthalmic division of the trigeminal nerve.

EXTERNAL LESIONS

- Neurofibromas (superficial tumors)
- Cafe-au-lait spots (macular hyperpigmentation)
- Axillary/inguinal freckling

BRAIN LESIONS

- Low-grade astrocytomas of the brainstem, tectum, and periaqueductal regions.
- Non-neoplastic hamartomatous lesions – non-enhancing, non-progressing lesions without any mass effect, and edema in basal ganglia (globus pallidus), optic radiations, WM, brainstem, and cerebral peduncles. The lesions may appear hyperintense on T1 and T2W. Foci of abnormal signal intensities (FSIs)/unidentified bright objects (UBOs) are also noted in adjacent WM.
- Arachnoid cyst in the middle cranial fossa.
- Prominent subarachnoid spaces.

OCULAR/ORBITAL LESIONS

- Optic nerve gliomas – can be bilateral, commonly extending into the optic chiasm, and even more posteriorly. They are hypo- to isointense on T1W and hyperintense on T2W.
- Ill-defined plexiform neurofibromas infiltrating the soft tissues of the eyelids, high deep masticator space, retrobulbar region, and

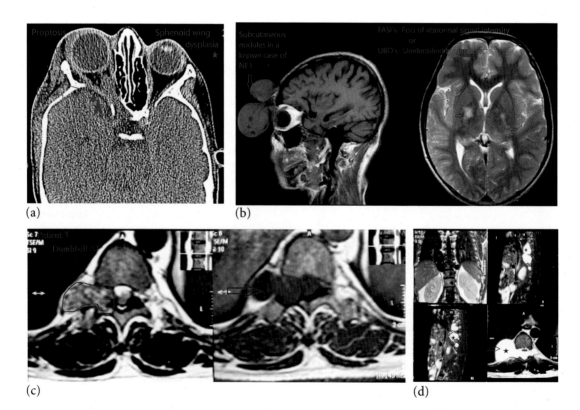

(a) (b) (c) (d)

Figure 8.1 (a) Sphenoid wing dysplasia, (b and c) subcutaneous nodules and T2W foci of high signal intensity in a patient with NF1, (c) dumbbell neurofibroma, and (d) lateral thoracic meningocele.

cavernous sinus. They appear isointense on T1W with intense contrast enhancement.
- Lisch nodules (pigmented iris hamartomas).
- Buphthalmos.

SPINAL CORD/NERVES
- Cord astrocytomas
- Non-neoplastic hamartomas of the cord
- Neurofibromas of the spinal nerves (dumbbell tumors)

OSSEOUS MANIFESTATIONS
- Sutural defects, mainly lambdoid sutures
- Hypoplastic greater wing of the sphenoid, with temporal herniation into the orbit
- Enlarged, empty orbit on the reformatted scan
- Enlargement of internal auditory canals, secondary to dysplastic, dural enlargement
- Enlarged neural foramina, usually secondary to neurofibroma along the exiting nerve root
- Meningoceles (lateral thoracic meningocele)
- Dural ectasia and dysplasia, with scalloping of posterior vertebral bodies and widened interpedicular distance
- Kyphoscoliosis
- Tibial bowing and pseudarthrosis
- Overgrowth of digit, ray, or limb
- Ribbon ribs
- Pectus excavatum/carinatum

VASCULAR LESIONS
- Progressive cerebral arterial occlusive disease with "moyamoya" pattern of occlusive disease
- Aneurysms
- Non-aneurysmal vascular ectasias
- Arteriovenous malformations

Neurofibromatosis Type 2

- Central type of NF with autosomal dominant inheritance and defects in chromosome 22.
- Less commonly involves the skin.
- MISME – multiple inherited schwannomas, meningiomas, and ependymomas.

BRAIN
- Multiple schwannomas of cranial nerves, especially the bilateral 8th cranial nerves followed by the trigeminal nerve
- Multiple meningiomas
- Non-neoplastic choroid plexus calcification

SPINE
- Multiple intradural, extramedullary schwannomas, or meningiomas
- Intramedullary ependymomas
- Secondary osseous changes, such as erosions and expansion

Segmental Neurofibromatosis

(NF-5) is a rare type that is associated with focal cutaneous and neural manifestations, e.g., lumbosacral plexus, scalp, etc. Patients present with pain and pruritus.

Tuberosus Sclerosis (TS, Bourneville Disease)

Autosomal dominant inheritance with a classic triad (EpiLoA) of:

1) **Epi**lepsy
2) **Lo**w intelligence
3) **A**denoma sebaceum (papular facial nevus)

BRAIN LESIONS
- *Cortical hamartomas/ tubers* are benign dysplastic foci of WM. They are visualized as hypodensities within broadened cortical gyri on a CT scan. They appear hyperintense on T1WI and hypointense on T2WI in neonates and young children (before myelination). In older children and adults, lesions appear isodense on CT scan; iso- to hypointense on T1W and hyperintense on T2WI.
- *WM lesions* along the lines of neuronal migration.
- *Subependymal nodules (SENs)* – benign lesions, seen as oval nodules protruding into the ventricles, with their long axis perpendicular to the ventricular wall. They are non-calcified in neonates and the tendency for calcification increases with age. Some of them may show contrast enhancement. Non-calcified lesions must be differentiated from subependymal heterotopias, which are non-enhancing, round to oval lesions, with their long axes in parallel to the ventricular surface. The lesions of heterotopia are isointense to gray matter on all pulse sequences.

  Calcified lesions must be differentiated from TORCH infection.

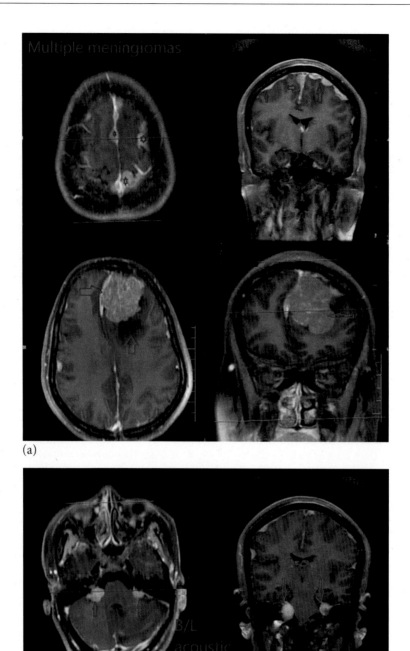

Figure 8.2 (a) Multiple meningiomas, and (b) bilateral acoustic schwannomas.

- *Subependymal giant cell astrocytoma (SEGAs/ SGCAs)* – calcified, heterogeneous, and intensely enhancing lesions that are located near the foramen of Monro, resulting in obstructive hydrocephalus.

ADDITIONAL LESIONS

- Retinal hamartomas
- Progressive occlusion of intracranial vessels
- Microcephaly
- Aneurysms

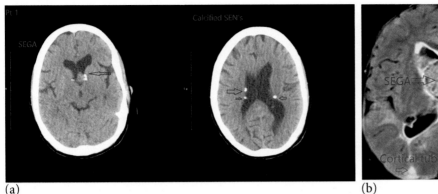

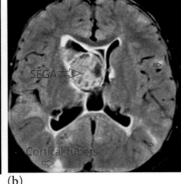

(a)   (b)

Figure 8.3 (a) SEGA and calcified subependymal nodules in a patient with TS, and (b) MRI findings of TS.

EXTRACRANIAL LESIONS

- Skin – facial angiofibromas, shagreen patches, hypomelanotic macules, subungual fibromas
- Heart – rhabdomyomas, aneurysms, vascular ectasias
- Kidneys – angiomyolipomas, renal cysts
- Musculoskeletal – bone islands, periosteal new bone
- Liver, spleen, pancreas – adenomas, leiomyomas
- Lungs – cystic lymphangioleiomyomatosis (LAM), fibrosis

Sturge-Weber Syndrome (Encephalotrigeminal Angiomatosis)

Persistent primitive venous plexus and impaired development of cortical venous drainage, leading to vascular congestion and hypoxia of the affected cortex.

CLINICAL

Seizures, dementia, hemiplegia, buphthalmos, vascular nevus (port wine stain) in the trigeminal nerve distribution.

IMAGING

The hallmark is unilateral cerebral atrophy and gyral pattern calcification.

CNS LESIONS

- Curvilinear gyral pattern calcifications, most prominent in the occipital and posterior parietal lobes on the same side as the facial angiomas
- Ipsilateral cerebral volume loss (hemiatrophy)

- Ipsilateral calvarial thickening and enlarged paranasal sinuses, mastoid, elevated petrous ridge due to progressive cortical hemiatrophy
- Enhancing pial angiomas
- Enhancement of ipsilateral choroid plexus from collateral venous drainage
- Prominent medullary and subependymal veins, with a paucity of normal cortical draining veins on MR venogram

NON-CNS LESIONS

- Congenital glaucoma
- Scleral telangiectasia and choroidal angiomas
- Vascular hyperplasia of oral mucosa and gingiva on the same side

MANAGEMENT

- Symptomatic treatment for seizures
- Cosmetic laser treatment
- Hemispherectomy

Von Hippel-Landau (VHL) Syndrome

Autosomal dominant lesion, characteristically with no skin involvement.

IMAGING

- Multiple hemangioblastomas (hypodense cystic lesion with avidly enhancing mural nodule) in cerebellum and spinal cord
- Retinal angiomas
- Multiple visceral cysts and tumors are noted in kidneys, pancreas, and liver
- Renal cell carcinoma > pheochromocytoma may be associated

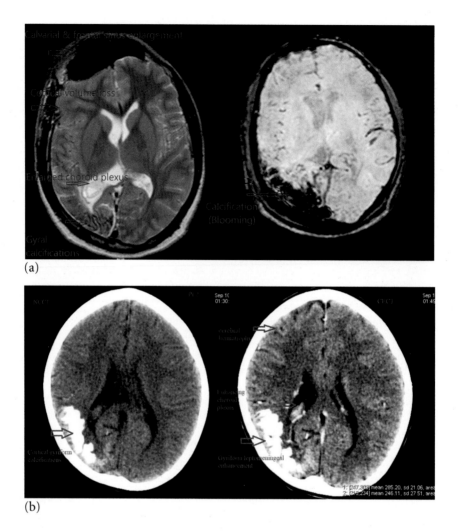

(a)

(b)

Figure 8.4 (a) MRI findings of SWS, and (b) CT findings of SWS.

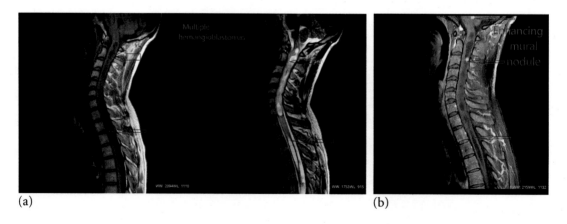

(a)   (b)

Figure 8.5 (a and b) Spinal and cerebellar hemangioblastomas in a patient with VHL.

- May be associated with bilateral endolymphatic sac tumors

DDs

Hemangioblastoma has to be differentiated from pilocytic astrocytoma (PA), which also presents as a cystic lesion with enhancing mural nodule, but the tumor nodule in PA lacks vascular flow voids and does not abut the pial or ependymal surface, as occurs in hemangioblastoma.

SUGGESTED READING

Nadgir, R, Yousem, DM. *Neuroradiology: The Requisites.* 4th ed. Philadelphia: Elsevier; 2017.

Osborn, AG, Salzman, KL, Jhaveri, MD, Barkovich, AJ. *Diagnostic Imaging: Brain.* Elsevier Health Sciences; 2015.

Watson, N, Watson, NA. *Jones H. Chapman & Nakielny's Guide to Radiological Procedures.* Elsevier; 2018.

9

Abnormal Skull

CONGENITAL LESIONS

- Dolichocephaly – abnormally long skull
- Brachycephaly – abnormally broad skull
- Bathrocephaly – occipital bone overlaps the parietal bone at the lambdoid suture, resulting in step-like deformity at the skull base

Lacunar Skull (Luckenschadel)

Finger-shaped rounded pits on the inner surface of the skull vault, that occur due to defects in the ossification of bones. It is usually associated with Chiari 2 malformation.

Sinus Pericranii

Small defect in the cranial vault, through which the transosseous emissary vein traverses. It results in abnormal communication between the extracranial venous structures and the intracranial dural sinuses, more prominent in the supine position than when sitting.

Intracranial Calcifications

- Tumors, like craniopharyngioma, gliomas, meningioma (amorphous), teratomas, chordomas, metastasis, and lipomas (marginal, bracket calcification)
- Infective lesions, like tuberculomas, neurocysticercosis, toxoplasmosis (basal ganglia linear streaks), cytomegalovirus (CMV, bilateral, and symmetrical periventricular), and paragonimus ("soap bubble" calcification in a cyst)
- Vascular lesions, like aneurysms (arc/ring-like) and chronic subdural hematomas

- Metabolic diseases, like hyperparathyroidism (falcine and tentorial), neurofibromatosis (choroid plexus), Sturge-Weber syndrome (gyral), tuberous sclerosis, and basal ganglia calcification in various etiologies, as described elsewhere in this book

Skull Erosions

NEOPLASTIC

- Bone tumors, like myelomas ("punched-out"/ "raindrop"), carcinomas ("moth-eaten"), dermoids, chordomas, leukemias, reticulosis, histiocytosis (geographic lesions with beveled edges), metastasis, and neuroblastoma (widened, irregular sutures)

NON-NEOPLASTIC

- Osteomyelitis, syphilis, and tuberculosis
- Post-traumatic erosions
- Neurofibromatosis, fibrous dysplasia
- Radiation necrosis, sarcoidosis
- Hyperparathyroidism ("pepper-pot skull")
- Osteoporosis circumscripta – well-delineated, lytic areas most commonly on frontal and occipital bones, affecting outer more than inner calvarial tables
- Parietal thinning – symmetrical, sharply-defined, localized thinning of outer table of parietal bones, commonly seen in elderly females

Hyperostosis

LOCALIZED

- Meningiomas

- Hyperostosis frontalis interna – bilaterally symmetrical, irregular thickening of the inner table of frontal bone, sparing the midline, commonly in post-menopausal females
- Osteomas (ivory nodules)
- Ossifying fibromas
- Fibrous dysplasia with leontiasis ossea (lion-like facies), affecting frontal and facial bones

GENERALIZED

- Acromegaly is associated with enlarged sinuses and prognathism
- Paget's disease – irregular, mottled texture of the skull vault
- Dystrophia myotonica – thickened skull vault with small pituitary fossa

Skull Base and Its Foramina

The skull base constitutes the floor of the cranial cavity, that divides the brain and facial components. Normally, it extends from the root of the nose anteriorly to the nuchal line posteriorly. It is composed of five bones: (1) paired frontal and temporal bones; (2) unpaired ethmoid, sphenoid and occipital bones. The base of the skull is divided into the anterior, middle, and posterior cranial fossae by the sphenoidal ridge anteriorly and the petrous ridge posteriorly. Neurovascular structures traverse through multiple foramina and canals visualized in the skull base.

The *anterior skull base*, comprising ethmoid and frontal bones, separates the anterior cranial fossa (ACF) from the paranasal sinuses and the orbits:

- Multiple small perforations in the cribriform plate of the ethmoid bone transmit olfactory nerves
- The anterior ethmoidal foramen transmits the anterior ethmoidal vessels and the nasociliary nerve
- The posterior ethmoidal foramen transmits the posterior ethmoidal vessels and nerve

APPLIED RADIOLOGY

Lesions involving ACF include sincipital encephalocele, benign sinonasal masses, such as polyps, hemangiomas, inverted papillomas, inflammatory mucosal disease, juvenile nasopharyngeal angiofibromas, and malignant masses, including sinonasal malignancy and olfactory neuroblastoma. Frontal bone osteomyelitis extends outward, forming a subgaleal abscess (Pott's puffy tumor), and is an infective lesion of the region. Traumatic fracture of the cribriform plate and the crista galli can result in CSF rhinorrhea.

The *central skull base*, mostly incorporating the sphenoid bone and the anterior part of the temporal lobe, constitutes the floor of the middle cranial fossa. The sella turcica (hypophyseal/pituitary fossa), in the body of the sphenoid bone, is bordered anteriorly by the tuberculum sellae and posteriorly by the dorsum sellae. The sphenoid sinus forms the floor of the sella. The diaphragma sellae, a dural fold, which is pierced by the pituitary stalk, forms the roof of the sella turcica. Its components are described below.

a) *Cavernous sinus* (CS)

Located on each side of the body of the sphenoid bone, the cavernous sinuses extend from the orbital apex and superior orbital fissure anteriorly to Meckel's cave (enclosing the trigeminal ganglion) and the petrous apex posteriorly. The internal carotid artery (ICA), surrounded by a sympathetic plexus and the abducens nerve (cranial nerve VI), lies in the central part of the CS. Cranial nerves III, IV and V (the ophthalmic and maxillary divisions) are located in the lateral dural wall of the CS, from superior to inferior. The CS connects the superior and inferior ophthalmic veins, the pterygoid plexus, and the Sylvian vein to the superior and inferior petrosal sinuses.

b) *Optic canal*

It is formed by the lesser wing of the sphenoid and transmits the optic nerve (cranial nerve II) and the ophthalmic artery.

c) *Superior orbital fissure (SOF)*

Bounded superiorly and inferiorly by the lesser and the greater wing of the sphenoid, respectively, the SOF allows transmission of various neurovascular structures like the oculomotor, trochlear, and abducens nerves; the first division of the trigeminal nerve, the orbital branch of the middle meningeal artery, various sympathetic filaments of the internal carotid plexus, the recurrent meningeal branches of the lacrimal artery, and the ophthalmic veins.

d) *Foramen rotundum*

Located in the base of the greater sphenoid wing, it is situated just inferolateral to the superior orbital fissure and joins the middle cranial fossa to the pterygopalatine fossa. The canal transmits the maxillary nerve (V2), the emissary veins and the artery of the foramen rotundum.

e) *Foramen ovale*

It lies posterolateral to the foramen rotundum in the posterior part of the sphenoid bone. It transmits the mandibular division of the trigeminal nerve [V$_3$], the lesser petrosal nerve, the accessory meningeal artery, and the emissary veins.

f) *Foramen spinosum*

It lies posterolateral to the foramen ovale in the greater wing of the sphenoid, and transmits the middle meningeal artery and the vein, and the recurrent branch of the mandibular nerve.

g) *Foramen lacerum*

This is not a real foramen and is filled with cartilage. Small meningeal branches of the ascending pharyngeal artery and emissary veins traverse through it. The greater petrosal nerve enters the posterolateral aspect and exits anteriorly as the nerve of the pterygoid canal. The carotid artery is not transmitted through the canal but rests on the endocranial aspect of the fibrocartilage.

h) *Vidian (pterygopalatine) canal*

It connects the pterygopalatine fossa anteriorly and the foramen lacerum posteriorly and is situated in the base of the pterygoid plates. It transmits the vidian artery (branch of the maxillary artery), and the vidian nerve (formed by the junction of the greater superficial petrosal nerve and the deep petrosal nerve)

i) *Pterygopalatine fossa (PPF)*

A pyramidal-shaped space, bounded anteriorly by the maxillary sinus, posteriorly by the pterygoid plates, and medially by the palatine bone. It contains the maxillary nerve, the pterygopalatine ganglion, and terminal branches of the internal maxillary artery.

j) *Carotid canal*

The internal carotid artery traverses the carotid canal, prior to its continuation as the middle cerebral artery, after which it runs across the circle of Willis to supply blood to the brain.

APPLIED RADIOLOGY

Fracture in the pterion, the weakest point in the skull, can damage the middle meningeal artery,

resulting in extradural hemorrhage. All the lesions involving the components mentioned above, the sellar, and the parasellar regions, are part of the CSB lesions.

The *posterior cranial fossa (PCF) or skull base (PSB)* is formed by the posterior part of the temporal bone and the occipital bone. Due to bone-induced beam-hardening artifacts on images, the evaluation of the PCF is often compromised.

a) The *foramen magnum*, part of occipital bone, is the largest foramen of the skull, which transmits vertebral arteries, anterior/posterior spinal arteries, and the spinal accessory nerve.

b) The *jugular foramen*, at the posterior end of the petro-occipital suture, is divided by a fibrous or bony septum into anteromedial pars nervosa and posterolateral pars vascularis. The right jugular foramen, being larger than the left in most of the population, is a normal variant, and occasionally both cranial nerves IX and X pass through the pars nervosa.

The *pars nervosa* is smaller than the pars vascularis, and the glossopharyngeal nerve (IX), with its tympanic branch (Jacobson's nerve), and the inferior petrosal sinus, are transmitted through it.

The *pars vascularis* is larger and the internal jugular vein, the vagus nerve (X), with its auricular branch (Arnold's nerve), the accessory nerve (XI), and the posterior meningeal artery, are transmitted through it.

c) The *hypoglossal canal* transmits the hypoglossal nerve (cranial nerve XII).

d) The *internal acoustic meatus* lies within the petrous part of the temporal bone (posteriorly). The facial nerve [VII], the vestibulocochlear nerve [VIII], and the labyrinthine artery traverse through it.

APPLIED RADIOLOGY

High-riding jugular bulb – the roof of the jugular bulb lies above the level of the floor of the internal auditory canal. It is more common on the right side and is a threatening variant that should be reported, especially before translabyrinthine surgery.

Paraganglioma and schwannoma are common lesions of the jugular foramen.

Clivus and petro-occipital fissure are common locations for chordomas and chondrosarcomas.

Meningioma, metastasis, multiple myeloma, and Langher cell histiocytosis can be seen anywhere in the skull base.

Cranial Nerves

Knowledge of the complicated anatomy of cranial nerves is pivotal to diagnosing various abnormalities involving the cranial nerves. High-resolution T2 CISS (constructive interference in steady-state) imaging helps in delineating the cranial nerves, especially in the cisterns and various foramen. Spread of a perineural tumor, which, if left undiagnosed, may worsen the prognosis, can be detected easily through thin-section post-Gadolinium T1 imaging.

OLFACTORY NERVE (CN I)

It consists of white matter (WM) tracts and lacks the layer of Schwann cells. It pierces the cribriform plate of the ethmoid bone, and then synapses in the olfactory bulb, finally ending in the temporal lobe, uncus, and entorhinal cortex. Airflow obstruction and mucosal atrophy due to chronic inflammation, tumors, or trauma may affect the sense of smell and result in anosmia.

OPTIC NERVE (CN II)

It is actually a brain tract (not a true cranial nerve) that is surrounded by subarachnoid space and myelinated by oligodendrocytes and not Schwann cells. Optic nerve has four parts: intraocular, intraorbital, intracanalicular, and intracranial (cisternal) segments. At the optic chiasm (termination of the optic nerve), the nasal fibers of each optic nerve decussate while the temporal fibers do not. From the optic chiasm arise two optic tracts, each one containing nasal fibers of the contralateral optic nerve and temporal fibers from the ipsilateral optic nerve. The optic tract courses around the cerebral peduncle to relay in the lateral geniculate body (LGB) of the thalamus, the axons of which constitute the optic radiations, enter the Meyer loop (around the inferior horns of the lateral ventricles), and then terminate in the calcarine cortex of the occipital lobe.

APPLIED RADIOLOGY

a) Globe or optic nerve pathology results in monocular visual loss.

b) Optic chiasm lesions (internal/external) result in bitemporal heteronymous hemianopsia, i.e., loss of both temporal visual fields.

c) Retrochiasmal pathology causes homonymous hemianopsia, i.e., vision loss that involves either the two right or the two left halves of both visual fields. A left-sided lesion causes right homonymous hemianopsia or *vice versa*.

d) In papilledema, the optic nerve head may appear elevated, the posterior sclera becomes flattened, and increased tortuosity, with dilatation of the perioptic subarachnoid spaces, may be noted.

e) Optic nerve tumors include gliomas and meningiomas. Gliomas appear as fusiform enlargement of the optic nerve, in comparison with irregular enlargement of the optic nerve sheath in meningiomas. Schwannomas and neurofibromas do not occur usually.

OCULOMOTOR NERVE (CN III)

It has both motor functions (innervate all the extraocular muscles except the superior oblique and the lateral rectus muscles) and parasympathetic functions (control pupillary sphincter function and accommodation). It has four segments:

a) The intra-axial segment is in the midbrain, just in front of the periaqueductal gray matter (GM).

b) The cisternal segment courses anteriorly toward the cavernous sinus, traversing between the posterior cerebral (PCA) and the superior cerebellar arteries (SCA).

c) The intracavernous segment runs along the lateral wall of the cavernous sinus.

d) The extracranial segment enters the orbit through the SOF and then divides into superior and inferior branches.

APPLIED RADIOLOGY

PCoA aneurysms often compress the cisternal segment of the 3rd nerve, causing pupil-involving 3rd nerve palsy. Pupil-sparing 3rd nerve palsy is commonly caused by microvascular infarction of the core of the nerve, with relative sparing of its peripheral fibers.

TROCHLEAR NERVE (CN IV)

It is a purely motor nerve, that innervates the superior oblique muscle, and is the only cranial nerve to exit the brainstem posteriorly. It also has four segments:

a) The intra-axial segment is in the midbrain, anterior to the periaqueductal GM, lying just below the oculomotor nerve nuclei.
b) The cisternal segment courses anteriorly in the ambient cistern and passes between the posterior cerebral and the superior cerebellar arteries.
c) The cavernous segment.
d) The extracranial segment that passes above the tendinous annulus of Zinn (CNs III and VI pass through the ring).

APPLIED RADIOLOGY

The long course and its close relationship to the tentorium make the trochlear nerve more susceptible to injury. Its palsy causes superior oblique paralysis, resulting in extorsion of the affected eye.

TRIGEMINAL NERVE (CN V)

The largest cranial nerve is a mixed sensory (major) and motor (minor) nerve that innervates the muscles of mastication. It also has four segments: a ganglion (the semilunar ganglion) and three postganglionic divisions.

a) The intra-axial segment has four nuclei (three sensory and one motor) that are located in the brainstem and the upper cervical spinal cord (between C2 and C4).
b) The cisternal segment.
c) The inter-dural segment lies entirely within the Meckel cave, where the nerve forms a mesh-like web, and, later, the Gasserian ganglion anteriorly before dividing.
d) The postganglionic segment of CN V consists of three divisions: CN V1 (the ophthalmic nerve), CN V2 (the maxillary nerve), and CN V3 (the mandibular nerve).

APPLIED RADIOLOGY

Denervation atrophy (shrinkage, fatty infiltration) of the muscles of mastication. Trigeminal neuralgia most often affects the maxillary and mandibular divisions. MR imaging is sensitive in delineating the compression by vascular structures.

ABDUCENS NERVE (CN VI)

It is a purely motor nerve and provides innervation to the lateral rectus muscle (abduction). It has five segments:

a) The intra-axial segment is located in the pons.
b) The cisternal segment lies in the prepontine cistern.
c) The inter-dural segment lies in the Dorello canal.
d) The cavernous segment exits the CS through the superior orbital fissure.
e) The intraorbital segment.

APPLIED RADIOLOGY

Intrinsic lateral rectus disease can mimic CN VI palsy. As a result of increased intracranial pressure, apical petrositis can cause abducens palsy.

FACIAL NERVE (CN VII)

It imparts motor innervation to the muscles of facial expression and taste sensation to the anterior two-thirds of the tongue. It also gives parasympathetic innervation to the lacrimal, submandibular, and sublingual glands.

It has six parts:

1) The intracranial (cisternal) segment.
2) The canalicular (meatal) segment courses through the cerebellopontine angle, together with the CN VIII, to the internal auditory canal.
3) The labyrinthine segment, the shortest and narrowest segment, has three branches, namely the greater superficial petrosal nerve, the lesser and the external petrosal nerve.
4) The tympanic segment.
5) The mastoid segment gives off the nerve to the stapedius and the chorda tympani nerve mainly.
6) The extratemporal segment; after exiting the skull at the stylomastoid foramen, it gives off motor branches, which supply the muscles of facial expression.

APPLIED RADIOLOGY

It is crucial to determine whether a facial nerve palsy is *central* (upper motor neuron type, due to a parenchymal lesion above the brainstem, that leads to the paralysis of the contralateral muscles of facial expression but spares the forehead) or *peripheral* (lower motor neuron type, that results in the paralysis of all ipsilateral muscles of facial expression].

Parotid malignancies, cerebellopontine angle (CPA) lesions like schwannomas, transverse temporal bone fractures, infective and inflammatory lesions like otitis media, reactivation of the herpes-zoster virus, cholesteatoma, Guillain-Barré syndrome, etc. can all afflict the facial nerve.

VESTIBULOCOCHLEAR NERVE (CN VIII)

This is a purely sensory nerve, which helps in hearing (cochlear nerve) and the sense of balance (vestibular nerve).

APPLIED RADIOLOGY

Vestibular schwannomas are most commonly seen in patients presenting with unilateral sensorineural hearing loss.

GLOSSOPHARYNGEAL NERVE (CN IX)

It is a sensory nerve specialized for taste sensation in the posterior third of the tongue. It also receives sensory fibers from the middle ear, pharynx, and viscerosensory fibers from the carotid body and sinus. It supplies motor fibers to the stylopharyngeus muscle and parasympathetic fibers to the parotid gland *via* the otic ganglion. Irritation of the nerve may result in glossopharyngeal neuralgia.

VAGUS NERVE (CN X)

It is a mixed nerve with motor (most of the soft palate, superior and recurrent laryngeal nerves), special (taste from the epiglottis), sensory (ear, larynx, viscera), and parasympathetic (regions of the head/neck, thorax, and abdominal viscera) functions. It leaves the skull through the jugular foramen (pars vascularis)

APPLIED RADIOLOGY

Head and neck tumors may cause recurrent laryngeal nerve (branch of the vagus nerve) palsy. Glomus tumors may result in vagal dysfunction.

SPINAL ACCESSORY NERVE (CN XI)

It is a purely motor nerve, that supplies the sternomastoid (aids head rotation) and trapezius muscles (helps in shrugging of shoulders). It may be injured during radical neck dissection.

HYPOGLOSSAL NERVE (CN XII)

It is a purely motor nerve that innervates both the intrinsic and most of the extrinsic muscles of the tongue. Any lesion of this nerve results in atrophy of the tongue muscles.

CASE STUDIES

Craniosynostosis (Craniostenosis, Sutural Synostosis, or Cranial Dysostosis)

Abnormal shape of the head is caused by premature obliteration of some cranial sutures, causing delay in growth and compensatory overgrowth at normal sutures. It can be non-syndromic (due to gene mutation) or syndromic (Apert syndrome, Waardenburg syndrome, or Carpenter syndrome), and may affect a single suture or multiple sutures.

Normal sutures allow skull growth perpendicular to their long axis, a phenomenon which is restricted in this pathology. The metopic suture closes first, followed by the coronal and lambdoid sutures. The sagittal suture is usually the last one to obliterate.

The sagittal suture is the single most common suture to be involved, followed by the coronal, metopic, lambdoid, and multiple sutures.

CLINICAL

Cosmetic disfigurement, neurological, and vascular compromise.

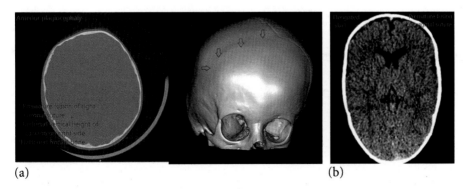

(a)   (b)

Figure 9.1 (a) Anterior plagiocephaly, (b) scaphocephaly.

IMAGING

CT with 3-D image reformatting is the best modality used for the evaluation of sutures. Associated brain anomalies can also be diagnosed.

DDs

Positional molding occurs due to external pressure post-delivery when an infant is placed in the same position for sleep for a long time.

MANAGEMENT

Cranioplasty.

ANCILLARY

- Scaphocephaly (boat-shaped skull) – premature fusion of sagittal sutures
- Trigonocephaly (triangular skull) – premature fusion of metopic suture
- Plagiocephaly (oblique/slanting skull) – premature fusion of lambdoid/coronal sutures unilaterally
- Brachycephaly – premature fusion of bilateral lambdoid/coronal sutures
- Oxycephaly (pointed skull)
- Acrocephaly (peak/summit skull)
- Turricephaly (tower skull)
- Cloverleaf skull (Kleeblattschadel) – most severe type and occurs due to intrauterine premature fusion of the sagittal, lambdoid, and coronal sutures (giving a trilobate shape like the clover)
- Harlequin eye – elevated superolateral corner of the orbit due to ipsilateral coronal suture synostosis

Persistent Metopic Suture (Metopism/Sutura Frontalis Persistans)

Also known as the frontal, interfrontal, or median frontal suture, it is a normal variant that runs through the midline from the nasion to the bregma across the frontal bone. Normally, its fusion starts at around three months of age and is completed by between nine months to two years of age.

CLINICAL

Asymptomatic.

IMAGING

- Radiolucent, irregular line with interdigitations, in the midline between the frontal bones
- Often associated with frontal sinus hypoplasia

DDs

Frontal bone fracture – not necessarily midline, look for associated soft tissue swelling and hematoma.

MANAGEMENT

No treatment required.

Frontoethmoidal (Sincipital) Encephalocele

Herniation of intracranial contents through a midline defect in the anterior cranial fossa. It can be

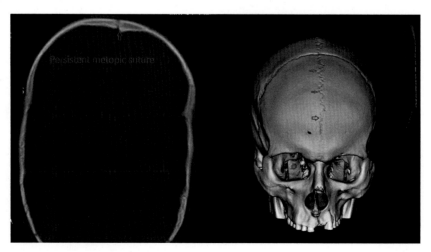

Figure 9.2 Persistent metopic suture.

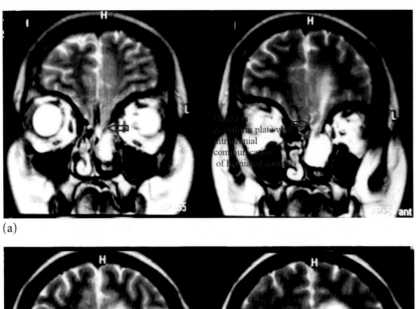

(a)

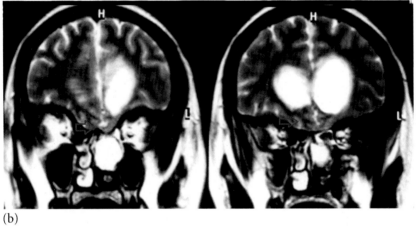

(b)

Figure 9.3 (a and b) Frontoethmoidal encephalocele.

the nasoethmoidal (most common type), naso-frontal, or naso-orbital type.

CLINICAL

Facial deformity, CSF rhinorrhea.

IMAGING

- NCCT – bony defect in cribriform plate, with soft tissue density in the nasal cavity extending intracranially
- MRI – intracranial communication, and the contents of the herniated sac are well delineated

DDs

- Traumatic encephalocele
- Frontoethmoid mucocele
- Polyps

MANAGEMENT

Surgery.

Bell's Palsy (Idiopathic Peripheral Facial Paralysis)

Usually idiopathic, but reactivation of the herpes simplex virus or the varicella-zoster virus, with latent infection in the geniculate ganglion, can also be a cause. It is rapid in onset but normally resolves in 6–8 weeks. The age range of presentation is usually 15–45 years. Risk factors are pregnancy, diabetes mellitus, and hypothyroidism.

CLINICAL

Sudden onset of facial weakness and altered taste sensation for a few days preceding paralysis, water

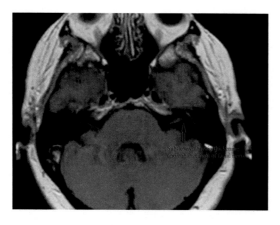

Figure 9.4 Facial nerve palsy.

drooling from the corner of the mouth, and weak eye closure.

IMAGING

Typical Bell's palsy does not require imaging. MRI to be considered if palsy is slow and progressive, associated with a spasm, recurrent in nature, or not showing signs of recovery after 6–8 weeks.

- High-resolution CT scan of the temporal bone – erosion and destruction of the facial nerve and its relationship with ossicles
- MRI – abnormal and asymmetric enhancement of cranial nerve exclude pathologies involving CPA or any other neoplasm compressing the nerve/any perineural spread

MANAGEMENT

- Self-resolving.

- Symptomatic treatment, like lubrication and patching for corneal dryness

Skull Base (Clival) Chordoma

A locally aggressive tumor that originates from embryonic remnants of the primitive notochord. Spheno-occipital, skull base or clival chordoma commonly occur in the 20–40 age group.

CLINICAL

Slow growing and presents as a result of mass effect on adjacent structures like the nasopharynx, brainstem, or cranial nerves.

IMAGING

- CT – destructive lytic lesion with an expansile soft-tissue mass in the midline, disproportionately large relative to the bony destruction, shows moderate to marked enhancement along with irregular intratumoral calcifications
- MRI – hypointense on T1W, hyperintense on T2W/ FLAIR, and heterogeneous enhancement with a "honeycomb" appearance
- GRE – blooming artifacts suggest variable intralesional calcifications/hemorrhages

DDs

Chondrosarcoma – chondroid matrix with rings and arc calcification, slightly off-midline, usually located in the thoracic vertebrae, and shows higher ADC values compared with clival chordoma.

MANAGEMENT

- Surgical resection
- Radiotherapy in recurrent cases

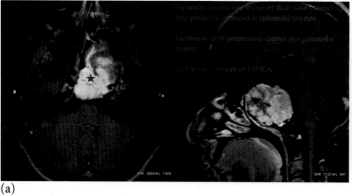
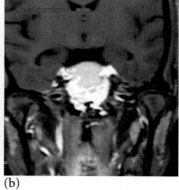

(a)

(b)

Figure 9.5 (a and b) MRI findings of clival chordoma.

SUGGESTED READING

Adam, A. *Grainger & Allison's Diagnostic Radiology: A Textbook of Medical Imaging.* Churchill Livingstone; 2008.

Bello, HR, Graves, JA, Rohatgi, S, Vakil, M, McCarty, J, Van Hemert, RL, Geppert, S, Peterson, RB. Skull base–related lesions at routine head CT from the emergency department: Pearls, pitfalls, and lessons learned. *Radiographics* 2019;39(4):1161–1182.

Romano, N, Federici, M, Castaldi, A. Imaging of cranial nerves: A pictorial overview. *Insights into Imaging* 2019;10(1):33.

Sheth, S, Branstetter, BF, Escott, EJ. Appearance of normal cranial nerves on steady-state free precession MR images. *Radiographics* 2009;29(4):1045.

10

Craniovertebral Junction Anomalies

The craniovertebral junction (CVJ) consists of:

- Occiput (posterior skull base)
- Atlas (first cervical vertebra C1)
- Axis (second cervical vertebra C2)
- Supporting ligaments

CRANIOMETRY

- The *Chamberlain line* (*palato-occipital line*) extends from the posterior pole of the hard palate to the opisthion (posterior margin of the foramen magnum). Normally, the tip of the odontoid process and the anterior arch of the atlas lie below this line.
- The *McGregor line* (*palatosuboccipital line*) extends between the posterior pole of the hard palate and the lowest point of the occipital squamosal surface.
- The *McRae line* (*foramen magnum line*) extends from the basion to the opisthion. Normally, the dens should not cross this line. Usually, the diameter of the foramen magnum is approximately 35–40 mm. Neurological symptoms may occur if this sagittal diameter is less than 19–20 mm.
- The *Wackenheim clivus baseline* (*basilar line*) extends along the clivus and extrapolates it inferiorly into the upper cervical spinal canal. The odontoid tip lies tangentially to the line and does not cross it.
- The *Welcher basal angle* is created at the junction of the nasion-tuberculum line and the tuberculum-basion line. Normally, it should be less than 140 degrees. This angle is increased in cases of platybasia and reduced to less than 130 degrees in achondroplasia.

- The *atlanto-occipital joint axis angle* is formed by lines drawn parallel to the atlanto-occipital joints. These lines intersect at the center of the odontoid process, with symmetrical condyles. A normal angle measures between 124 and 127 degrees, which may become more obtuse in the presence of occipital condyle hypoplasia.

MRI superbly delineates the ligaments that connect the occipital bone and the cervical vertebrae, along with achieving the stability and flexibility of the CVJ.

The flexion and extension of the cervical spine occur at the atlanto-occipital joint between the occipital condyles and the lateral masses of C1. Cervical rotation mainly occurs at the atlantoaxial articulation between the lateral masses of C1 and C2.

External Craniocervical Ligaments

- *Anterior atlanto-occipital membrane* – around 2 cm wide, intermediate signal intensity, densely woven structure that extends from the upper aspect of the anterior arch of Cl to the foramen magnum. It is continuous caudally with the anterior atlantoaxial ligament and then to the anterior longitudinal ligament (ALL) of the spinal column.
- *Posterior atlanto-occipital membrane* – a structure which is wavy, less strong, and with low signal intensity, extending from the posterior arch of Cl to the foramen magnum. Its apertures allow passage of the vertebral arteries, accompanying veins and cranial nerves.
- *Lateral atlanto-occipital ligaments* – oriented vertically.

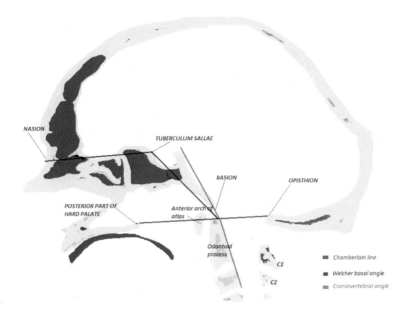

Figure 10.1 Craniometry of CVJ.

- *Interspinous ligaments* – oblique orientation; seen as several separate fibers of intermediate signal on midline images.

Internal Craniocervical Ligaments

- *Tectorial membrane* – superior extension of the posterior longitudinal ligament (PLL), which attaches to the anterolateral aspect of the foramen magnum. This low-signal, strong ligament is pivotal for limiting flexion.

- *Transverse ligament* – thick, strong, intermediate-signal band, oriented in the coronal plane, extending from a tubercle on the inner part of one side of the atlas to a tubercle on the opposite side. The transverse ligament and its fasciculi have a cross shape and together constitute the cruciform ligament. It limits anterior translation and flexion of the atlanto-axial joints.

- *Apical ligament* – not directly visible on MR or anatomic sections. It lies superior to the dens, extending to the occipital bone, and is

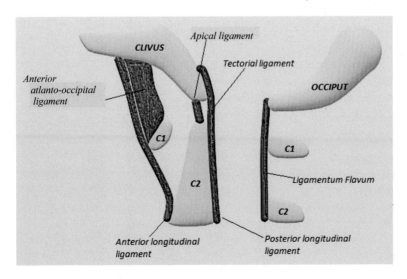

Figure 10.2 Various craniocervical ligaments.

surrounded by fat. It lies between the superior longitudinal fasciculus of the cruciform ligament and the anterior atlanto-occipital membrane.

- *Alar ligaments* – strong, broad structures with intermediate signal intensity. They extend outward from the superior and lateral aspect of the dens to the medial aspect of the occipital condyle. They allow anterior shift of C1 from 3–5 mm and strengthen the atlanto-occipital capsule. These limit axial rotation and side bending, while allowing flexion and extension.

Anomalies of Occiput

CONDYLUS TERTIUS (THIRD OCCIPITAL CONDYLE)

A tiny separate ossicle, anteromedial to the occipital condyle, is noted when the proatlas (fourth occipital sclerotome) fails to integrate. It may form a joint/pseudo joint, with the odontoid process or with the anterior arch of the atlas restricting the range of motion of the CVJ.

CONDYLAR HYPOPLASIA

Underdeveloped/flattened occipital condyles, leading to basilar invagination and widening of the atlanto-occipital joint axis angle.

HYPOPLASIA OF THE BASIOCCIPUT

This results in clival shortening and is associated with basilar invagination.

ATLANTO-OCCIPITAL ASSIMILATION/ OCCIPITALIZATION OF THE ATLAS

This occurs due to failure of segmentation between the skull and the first cervical vertebra. It may be complete or partial and leads to basilar invagination. The clivus-canal angle may be reduced, though the Wackenheim clivus baseline may be normal.

Anomalies of Atlas

- *Posterior rachischisis*
- *Clefts of the atlas arches,* usually midline
- *Posterior atlas arch aplasia (total/partial)* is rare
- *Anterior arch rachischisis*
- *Split atlas* denotes anterior and posterior arch rachischisis

- *Ponticle* – calcification/ossification along the margins of the foramen on the atlanto-occipital ligament. It can be posterior or lateral.

Anomalies of Axis

- *Persistent ossiculum terminale (Bergman ossicle)* results from the failure of fusion of the terminal ossicle to the remainder of the odontoid process. Normally, the fusion occurs by 12–13 years of age. Sometimes, it may mimic a type 1 odontoid fracture (avulsion of the terminal ossicle) and needs differentiation.
- *Total aplasia of the odontoid process*
- *Os odontoideum*

Congenital Malformations

These include Chiari malformations, achondroplasia, osteogenesis imperfecta, Down syndrome, mucopolysaccharidoses, etc.

KLIPPEL-FEIL SYNDROME

Faulty segmentation of cervical somites, resulting in vertebral fusion.

Classic triad of:

- Low posterior hairline
- Short neck
- Limited neck motion

It is associated with Sprengel's deformity, scoliosis, cardiac, pulmonary, and genitourinary conditions.

Acquired Disorders

Degenerative arthritis, rheumatoid arthritis (laxity of transverse and alar ligaments), and other infectious, inflammatory, and neoplastic etiologies.

Trauma

FLEXION INJURIES

- Simple wedge fracture with intact posterior ligaments
- Anterior subluxation (hyperflexion sprain) due to the rupture of posterior ligaments
- Unstable wedge fracture, with damage to both the anterior column (anterior wedge fracture)

and the posterior column (interspinous ligament)
- Unilateral and bilateral interfacet dislocation ("teardrop" fracture)

EXTENSION INJURIES

- Anterior atlantoaxial dislocation
- Hangman's fracture
- Traumatic spondylolisthesis of C2
- Extension teardrop fracture of C2

Jefferson burst fracture of the C1 ring with lateral displacement of both articular masses.

LATERAL FLEXION INJURIES

- Uncinate process fracture
- Transverse process fracture
- Unilateral occipital condylar fracture
- Unilateral fracture, lateral mass, C1

MISCELLANEOUS

- Occipitoatlantal dissociation
- Odontoid fractures
- Torticollis
- Atlantoaxial rotatory dissociation

Atlanto-occipital dislocation – marked flexion or extension at the upper cervical level result in complete disruption of all the ligaments between the occiput and the atlas, with immediate death ensuing from stretching of the brainstem (respiratory arrest). Cervical traction is contraindicated.

ATLANTOAXIAL SUBLUXATION

Predental space – distance between the anterior dens and posterior tubercle of the atlas (C1); usually <3 mm in adults and <5 mm in children
     Normally, the transverse ligament restricts the forward movement of the atlas on the axis.

ETIOLOGY

- Trauma
- Rheumatoid arthritis – laxity/disruption of the transverse ligament with articular cartilage destruction, pannus formation, and odontoid erosion
- Down syndrome – lax transverse ligament
- Grisel syndrome – associated with inflammation of adjacent soft tissues of the neck
- Retro-odontoid pseudotumor – non-neoplastic T2-hyperintense mass due to degeneration of transverse ligament

IMAGING

- Increased predentate space
- Spinal canal anteroposterior diameter at C2 <18 mm
- Disruption of spinolaminar lines

OCCIPITAL CONDYLE FRACTURE

Vertical compression and lateral bending.
     Associated with head trauma, accompanied by cranial nerve deficits.

BASILAR INVAGINATION

A primary developmental anomaly in which the abnormally high vertebral column becomes prolapsed into the skull base. It may be associated with basiocciput hypoplasia, occipitalization, Klippel-Feil syndrome, Chiari malformations, and atlanto-occipital assimilation.

CLINICAL

Headache, dizziness, numbness, paralysis.

IMAGING

- Tip of odontoid
     >3 mm above the Chamberlain line
     >4.5 mm above the McGregor line
     >5 mm above the McRae line
- Shortening of basiocciput

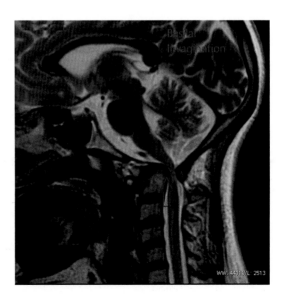

Figure 10.3 Basilar invagination.

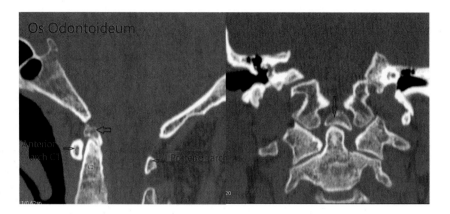

Figure 10.4 Os odontoideum.

- Short and horizontally oriented clivus
- May be associated with *platybasia* – flattening of the skull base, manifested by an increase in the Welcher basal angle

DDs

- Basilar impression – secondary or acquired form of basilar invagination due to softening of the skull base, in association with Paget's disease, Hurler syndrome, rickets, skull base infection, osteomalacia, hyperparathyroidism, and osteogenesis imperfecta

MANAGEMENT

Surgery.

Os ODONTOIDEUM

From birth until the age of eight years, the odontoid base is separated from the body of the axis by cartilage, which becomes ossified later or may remain segregated as an independent structure lying above the axis body (in the position of the odontoid process), resulting in cruciate ligament incompetence and atlantoaxial instability.

Imaging and DDs

See Table 10.1.

Ancillary

Two types:

- Orthotopic – normal position with a broad gap between the os odontoideum and C2
- Dystopic – displaced position near the skull base

ODONTOID FRACTURE

Anderson and D'Alonzo Classification:

- Type 1 – avulsion of the tip of the dens at the attachment of the alar ligament
  - Stable and rare
- Type 2 – fracture through the base of the dens
  - Unstable and the most frequent type

Table 10.1 Comparison between Os Odontoideum and Type 2 Odontoid Fracture

	Os Odontoideum	Type 2 Odontoid Fracture
Upper margin of axis body	Well-corticated/sclerotic, smooth, and convex	Flattened, sharp, irregular, and nonsclerotic/uncorticated
Anterior arch of atlas	Hypertrophic and rounded	Normal half-moon-shaped appearance
Location relative to superior articular facet	Above	Below
Odontoid orientation	Vertical	Maybe tilted

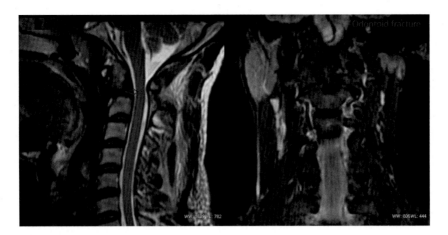

Figure 10.5 MRI findings of an odontoid fracture.

- Type 3 – fracture through the body of the axis
  - Unstable but has better prognosis

CLINICAL

Pain, unstable neck, quadriplegia.

IMAGING AND DDs

See Table 10.1.

SUGGESTED READING

Adam, A. *Grainger & Allison's Diagnostic Radiology: A Textbook of Medical Imaging.* Churchill Livingstone; 2008.

Osborn, AG, Salzman, KL, Jhaveri, MD, Barkovich, AJ. *Diagnostic Imaging: Brain.* Elsevier Health Sciences; 2015.

Riascos, R, Bonfante, E, Cotes, C, Guirguis, M, Hakimelahi, R, West, C. Imaging of atlanto-occipital and atlantoaxial traumatic injuries: What the radiologist needs to know. *Radiographics* 2015;35(7):2121–2134.

11

Congenital Anomalies

NORMAL ANATOMY

The neural tube is formed by the longitudinal closure of the neural plate, the upper part forming the brain and the lower part forming the spinal canal, as discussed in Chapter 1. A defect in this closure results in dysraphism.

The spinal cord is developed in three main stages – gastrulation, primary neurulation, and secondary neurulation during early embryogenesis.

- Gastrulation (second or third week) – conversion of the embryonic bilaminar disk to a trilaminar disk, composed of the ectoderm, the mesoderm, and the endoderm. The notochord is formed from the midline mesoderm interacting with the overlying ectoderm.
- Primary neurulation (third or fourth week) – formation of the neural plate and eventually the closure of the neural tube in a zip-like manner.
- Secondary neurulation (fifth or sixth week) – formation of the central canal (canalization), with the caudal cell mass undergoing retrogressive differentiation to form the conus medullaris, filum terminale, ventriculus terminalis, and most of the sacrum and coccyx.

Spinal dysraphism results from defective primary neurulation, whereas defective secondary neurulation results in filar lipoma, tight filum terminale, caudal agenesis, and sacrococcygeal teratoma.

Apart from this, complex dysraphic states include disorders of midline notochordal integration (neurenteric cysts and diastematomyelia) and disorders of notochordal formation (caudal regression syndrome and segmental spinal dysgenesis).

LIPOMYELOCELE

A type of closed/occult spinal dysraphism and a disorder of primary neurulation, where premature dysjunction leads to entrapment of mesenchymal tissue into the spinal canal. Depending on the timing of dysjunction, the lipomatous spectrum of spinal dysraphism can include those shown in Figure 11.1.

CLINICAL

Hairy nevus, mole, dimples (>2.5 cm from the anal verge), pseudo tail, lipoma, hemangioma, and aplasia cutis/dermal sinus. It can rarely present as a bowel/bladder dysfunction.

IMAGING

- CT – subcutaneous fat continuous with the spinal canal by posterior dysraphism
  - Focal widening of the bony spinal canal
- MRI – defect in sacral vertebrae, with herniation of subcutaneous fat within the spinal canal
  - The neural lipoma-placode interface lies *within* the spinal canal (best visualized on T1WI)
  - Skin overlying the defect may show subcutaneous fat hypertrophy

DDs

- Lipomeningomyelocele
- Intraspinal (intradural) lipoma – no associated dysraphism, and the overlying dura is intact

ANCILLARY

Commonly associated with syringomyelia and vertebral segmentation anomalies.

Placode is frequently rotated to one side and can cause stretch injury to nerve roots.

Table 11.1 Comparison of Open and Closed Spinal Dysraphism

Open Spinal Dysraphism	Closed Spinal Dysraphism
Cord and its covering are exposed to the outside	Neural elements of the cord are not exposed
No skin or mesenchymal tissue covers the sac	Skin or mesenchymal elements cover the sac
Examples include myelocele and myelomeningocele	It can occur with or without subcutaneous mass. Examples include dorsal dermal sinus, lipomyelomeningocele, terminal myelocystocele, filar lipoma, tight filum terminale, etc.

DIASTEMATOMYELIA

Involves complete or partial clefting of the cord, usually occurring between D9 and S1 level, and presents in childhood, with a higher frequency in females. Affected infants commonly present with a hairy tuft of skin, hemangioma, nevus, or pilonidal cyst on the skin of the back.

CLINICAL

Motor or sensory weakness, involving the lower extremities, bowel or bladder dysfunction, gait abnormalities, or scoliosis.

Pang Classification of split cord malformation.

IMAGING

- CT – better for fibrous bands and non-marrow-containing bony spicules

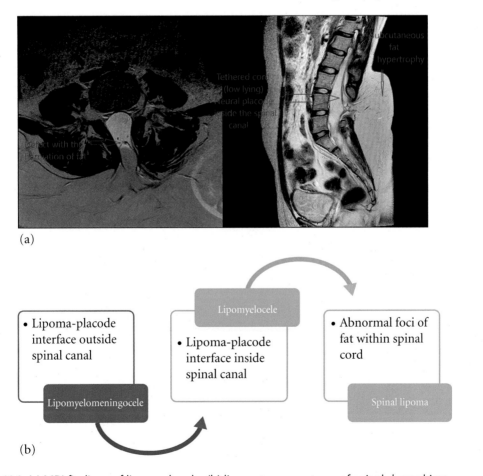

(a)

(b)

Figure 11.1 (a) MRI findings of lipomyelocele, (b) lipomatous spectrum of spinal dysraphism.

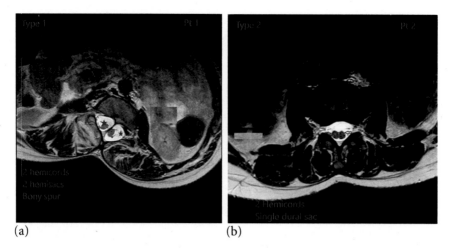

(a)   (b)

Figure 11.2 (a) Type 1 diastematomyelia, (b) Type 2 diastematomyelia.

Table 11.2 Comparison of Type 1 with Type 2 Diastematomyelia

Type 1	Type 2
Two hemicords with two spinal canals and two dural sacs	Two hemicords with a single spinal canal and a single dural sac
Osseous spur	Fibrous bands
More commonly symptomatic	Usually asymptomatic, unless associated with tethering or hydromyelia

- MRI – better for fibrocartilaginous and marrow-containing bony spicules

DDs

- Dimyelia – duplicated spinal cord
- Diplomyelia – accessory spinal cord

MANAGEMENT

Treatment consists of surgical tethered cord release, spur resection, scoliosis correction, and dural repair.

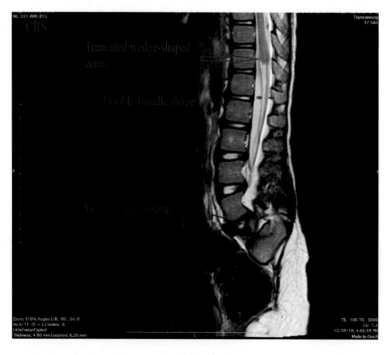

Figure 11.3 Imaging findings of caudal regression syndrome.

CAUDAL REGRESSION SYNDROME

Rare anomaly of caudal spine and spinal cord, more common in male infants of diabetic mothers.

CLINICAL

Sensory deficits, short intergluteal cleft, atrophy of distal musculature.

IMAGING

- Caudal lumbar/sacrococcygeal agenesis/hypogenesis
- Truncated spinal cord terminating above the expected level
- Wedge-shaped conus medullaris
- Double-bundle contour – abnormal course of cauda equina, with separation of the anterior and posterior nerve roots
- Spinal canal narrowing rostral to the last intact vertebra
- Associated with vertebral defects, tethered cord, lipomas, orthopedic, and genitourinary anomalies

DDs

- Sirenomelia (mermaid syndrome) – severe caudal dysgenesis with fused lower extremities
- Lipomyelomeningocele

MANAGEMENT

Symptomatic.

SUGGESTED READING

Adam, A. *Grainger & Allison's Diagnostic Radiology: A Textbook of Medical Imaging.* Churchill Livingstone; 2008.

Osborn, AG, Salzman, KL, Jhaveri, MD, Barkovich, AJ. *Diagnostic Imaging: Brain.* Elsevier Health Sciences; 2015.

Rufener, SL, Ibrahim, M, Raybaud, CA, Parmar, HA. Congenital spine and spinal cord malformations—Pictorial review. *American Journal of Roentgenology* 2010;194(3):S26–S37.

12

Acquired Diseases

NORMAL ANATOMY

The normal spine, with an "S" curve, when viewed from the side, is divided into five sections:

- Cervical – seven vertebral segments, eight nerve roots
- Thoracic – 12 vertebral segments, 12 nerve roots
- Lumbar – five vertebral segments, five nerve roots
- Sacral – five fused segments, five nerve roots
- Coccygeal – four rudimentary vertebrae

At each level, a spinal nerve root, with specific motor and sensory functions, leaves the spinal cord. The white matter in the periphery and the central gray matter give it a butterfly shape.

Ligaments

- The anterior longitudinal ligament (ALL) extends from the basiocciput to S1, and connects the anterior portion of the vertebral bodies with one another
- The posterior longitudinal ligament (PLL) extends from C1 to the first sacral vertebra and connects the posterior portion of the vertebral bodies
- The ligamentum flavum joins the lamina of adjoining levels
- Interspinous ligaments connect the neighboring spinous processes

The spine should be evaluated by three curved, roughly parallel lines:

1) The ALL line follows the anterior border of the vertebral bodies

2) The PLL line follows the posterior border of the vertebral bodies
3) The spinolaminar line follows the anterior border of the posterior spinous processes, where the laminae converge

Cervical Spine

C1 (Atlas) does not have a vertebral body but has a bony ring formed of anterior and posterior arches, which are connected by lateral masses on either side. The ellipsoid superior articular surface combines with the occipital joint to form the atlanto-occipital joint, and the round inferior articular surface combines with superior facets of the C2 vertebra to form the atlantoaxial joints.

C2 (Axis) supports C1 and allows for rotation at the C1–C2 joint. The dens or odontoid process is a superior projection that articulates with the anterior arch of C1.

C3–C7 are described below.

ANTERIOR ELEMENTS

- Box-shaped vertebral bodies with uncovertebral joints
- Intervertebral disc space (IVDS) with central nucleus pulposus and peripheral annulus fibrosus
- Transverse processes and foramina transversaria containing vertebral arteries and veins

POSTERIOR ELEMENTS

- Pedicles that connect vertebral bodies to articular pillars
- Articular pillars and facet joints (synovial joints with a fibrous capsule)
- Laminae are thin bony plates, fused in the midline, and which cover the spinal canal

- Spinous processes are usually bifid. C7 has the longest spinous process

SPINAL CANAL

- Anteroposterior vertebrae vary from 15–16 mm at the cervical level to ~12 mm at the lumbar level

Foramen transversarium and the uncinate process are exclusive to the cervical spine. Other ligaments in the cervical region have been described in Chapter 11 (CV junction).

Thoracolumbar Spine

T1 is the first rib bearing a vertebral segment, and T12 is the last rib bearing a vertebral segment.

The spinal cord terminates between T12 and L2. Cauda equina (horsetail) refers to the nerve roots below the spinal cord collectively.

It is composed of:

- Anterior elements – vertebral bodies and intervertebral discs
- Posterior elements – pedicles, articular pillars, laminae, spinous processes, and facet joints
- Ligaments (low signal intensity [SI])
- Epidural fat, venous plexus (interposed between PLL and the vertebral body)
- Neural tissue – conus medullaris, cauda equina, sacral plexus, lumbar roots and nerves

MRI Features

- Red (hematopoietically active and cellular) or yellow (inactive and fatty) marrow can be differentiated on MRI.

- In young children (<7 years), red marrow is seen predominantly, that appears isointense on T1W. Moderate to intense enhancement is noted up to two years of age, which fades gradually and disappears by the age of seven years.
- From the age of seven to adolescence, progressive conversion to yellow marrow is noted, resulting in heterogeneous (due to focal fat deposition) high SI on T1W and low SI on T2WI. No contrast enhancement is seen, even in adults.

SI OF INTERVERTEBRAL DISCS (IVDs)

Infants have high SI on T2WI, with a central low SI area of the notochord remnant.

Adults have hyperdense IVD on non-enhanced CT. The outer annulus is low SI on T1W and T2W. The nucleus pulposus is high SI on T2WI.

Spinal Lesions

See Figure 12.1 and Table 12.1.

Case Studies

Disc Herniation with Extrusion

Commonly affects the lumbosacral spine at the L4-L5/L5-S1 levels.

CLINICAL

Backache, radiculopathy.

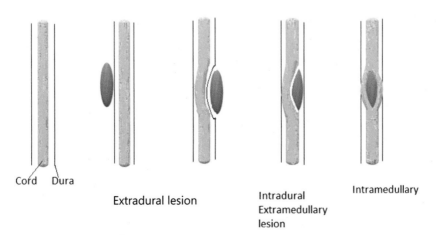

Cord   Dura

Extradural lesion

Intradural Extramedullary lesion

Intramedullary

Figure 12.1 Diagrammatic representation of extradural and intradural spinal lesions.

Table 12.1 Comparison of Extradural, Intradural Extramedullary, and Intradural Intramedullary Lesions

Extradural	Intradural Extramedullary	Intradural Intramedullary
• Compression with the displacement of the cord away from the mass • Narrowing of the ipsilateral and contralateral subarachnoid space (SAS)	• Displacement of the spinal cord away from the mass • Enlarged ipsilateral and effaced contralateral CSF space surrounding the mass • Erosion of neural foramen • Filling defect with meniscus sign	• Expansion of the spinal cord with irregularity • Narrowing of the adjacent SAS
• Metastasis • Disc herniation, epidural abscess, hematoma	• Tumors (meningioma, schwannoma, neurofibroma)	• Tumors (ependymoma, astrocytoma, hemangioblastoma) • Vascular lesions • Cord infarct, multiple sclerosis, transverse myelitis

IMAGING

- CT – osteophytes
  - Vacuum phenomenon – nitrogen gas within the disc space and herniated disc
- MRI – focal herniation of low to intermediate SI disc which may cause cord compression
  - Disc migration – caudal or cephalad
  - T2 high SI annular tear
  - Spinal canal narrowing due to disc bulge, ligamentum flavum hypertrophy, and facet arthrosis
  - Nerve compression may occur at the level of disc, lateral recess, foraminal, and extraforaminal
- CEMRI – peripheral enhancement caused due to inflammation with non-vascularized, non-enhancing material within the extruded material
- MR myelography – cut-off if extrusion causes spinal stenosis

MANAGEMENT

Anti-inflammatory medication/surgery.

Vertebral Hemangioma

Benign vascular lesions frequently noted in thoracolumbar spine, common in females, and frequency increases with age. Rarely, they can present as a locally aggressive vertebral hemangioma.

CLINICAL

Asymptomatic; severe pain should point toward the possibility of vertebral collapse.

IMAGING

CT:

- Decreased attenuation of the vertebral body due to the presence of fatty marrow, intermixed with thickened bony trabeculae
- Classic "polka dot" appearance on axial and "corduroy" appearance on sagittal CT images, due to trabecular thickening

MRI:

- Lesion appears hyperintense on T1 (intralesional fat) and T2WI (high water content), with marked post-contrast enhancement (highly vascular)

DDs

- Metastasis – hypointense on T1WI and hyperintense on T2WI. Atypical hemangiomas may be difficult to differentiate from metastasis.

MANAGEMENT

Asymptomatic; no treatment required.

Marked pain or nerve compression symptoms – balloon kyphoplasty, radiotherapy, or laminectomy with transarterial embolization.

Pott's Spine (Tuberculous Spondylitis)

The most common form of skeletal involvement in tuberculosis spreads by hematogenous seeding of the vertebral body. Radiographic features are often quite advanced as the infection is indolent in nature.

CLINICAL

Fever, night sweats, weight loss, severe backache, lower limb weakness/paraplegia, and kyphotic deformity.

Raised ESR and positive sputum for AFB (acid-fast bacilli).

IMAGING

CT:

- Vertebral height reduction with endplate irregularity
- Classic sparing of intervertebral disc
- Wedge compression of anterior vertebral body, causing Gibbus deformity
- Irregularity of anterior vertebral margin due to subligamentous spread
- Paravertebral opacification due to abscess
- Ivory vertebra and vertebra plana in late stages

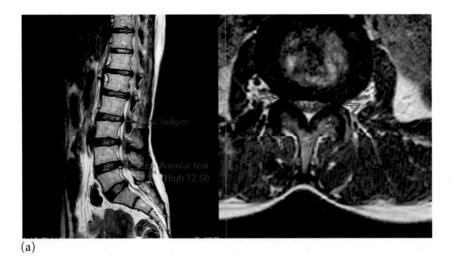

(a)

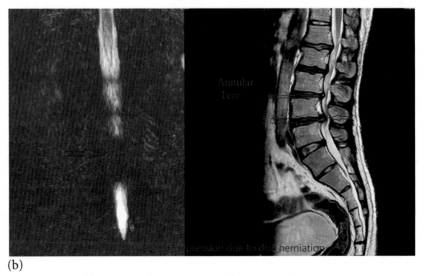

(b)

Figure 12.2 (a) Annular tear with disc bulges and ligamentum flavum hypertrophy, (b) complete cut-off due to disc herniation and annular tear with disc herniation.

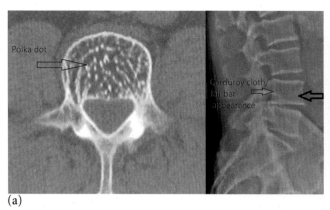
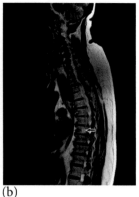

(a) (b)

Figure 12.3 (a and b) Imaging findings of vertebral hemangioma.

MRI:

- Marrow appears hypointense on T1W, hyperintense on T2W
- Well-circumscribed paraspinal/psoas collection/abscess
- CEMRI – shows post-contrast marrow and subligamentous enhancement. Abscess enhances peripherally with fluid intensity center

DDs

- Metastasis – posterior vertebral body, pedicles, and laminar involvement favors metastasis
- Brucellosis – lumbar spine involvement is more common

MANAGEMENT

- Systemic antitubercular regimen
- Palliative therapy – analgesics
- Percutaneous drainage of abscess with antibiotic cover

ANCILLARY

Concurrent pulmonary tuberculosis/history of prior infection to be evaluated.

Associated psoas abscess and calcification of paraspinal lesions are characteristic.

Transverse Myelitis

An inflammatory pathology of the spinal cord, which may be idiopathic or have certain underlying etiologies – post-infection (usually viral or acute disseminated encephalomyelitis [ADEM]), autoimmune diseases, or resulting from systemic malignancy.

CLINICAL

Paresis, sphincter dysfunction.

IMAGING

CT and MRI:

- Involves >3–4 spinal cord segments
- Involvement of >2/3 of the cross-sectional area
- Thoracic cord most frequently involved
- Cord expansion
- Poorly delineated T2-hyperintense lesions, predominantly central spinal cord
- Variable post-contrast enhancement patterns

DDs

- Multiple sclerosis – lesions involve <50% of the cross-sectional area, fewer than two vertebral body segments, and are peripherally located. The brain may show characteristic Dawson's fingers.
- ADEM – younger age at presentation, and monophasic disease course.
- Spinal cord infarct.
- Intramedullary neoplasm.

MANAGEMENT

Treat underlying etiology.

Burst Fractures

Compression fractures eventuating as a result of high-intensity axial loading – fall from a height, and mostly involving thoracolumbar spine.

CLINICAL

Backache, sensory, or motor deficit.

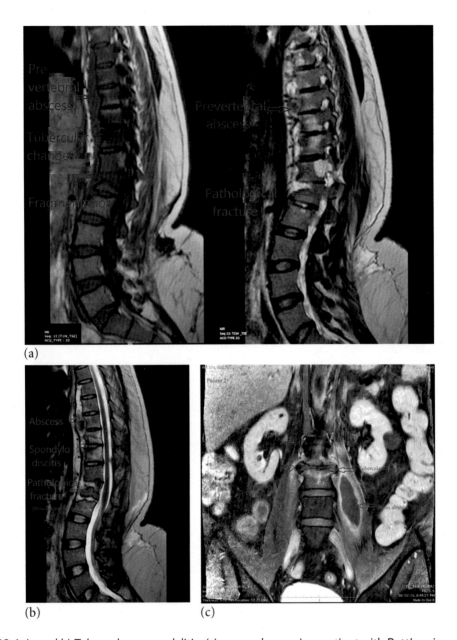

Figure 12.4 (a and b) Tuberculous spondylitis, (c) psoas abscess in a patient with Pott's spine.

IMAGING

CT:

- Decreased vertebral height, with comminuted fracture of the involved vertebrae
- Retropulsion of bony fragments posteriorly into the spinal canal, compressing/injuring the cord
- Interpedicular widening

MRI:

- Spinal cord edema/ contusion/ transection

DDs

- Wedge compression fracture
- Degenerative osteoporotic fractures
- Chance fracture

MANAGEMENT

Depends on severity – conservative/surgery.

Table 12.2 Differentiation between Pyogenic and Tubercular Discitis

Pyogenic Discitis	Tubercular Discitis
Involves disc spaces	Spares disc spaces until late stages
Lumbar spine	Thoracic spine
Single level	Multilevel involvement
Less bony destruction, but extensive inflammation	Extensive bone destruction
Thick, irregular abscess wall	Thin, smooth abscess wall

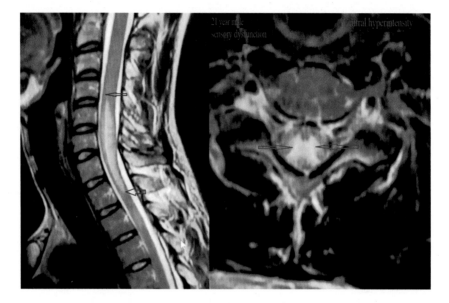

Figure 12.5 Imaging findings of transverse myelitis.

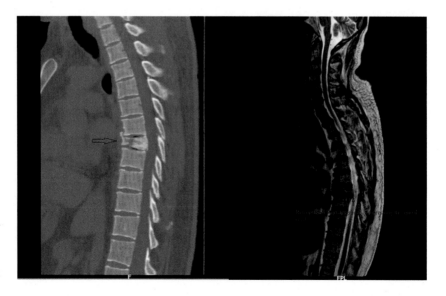

Figure 12.6 Imaging findings of burst fracture.

Spondylolisthesis

Slipping/displacement/subluxation of one vertebra relative to a lower one. It can be congenital, traumatic, degenerative, or due to any pathological etiology.

CLINICAL

Backache.

IMAGING

- Anterolisthesis – anterior slippage
- Retrolisthesis – backward slippage

Grading

Grade 1 – displacement <25%
Grade 2 – displacement 25–50%
Grade 3 – displacement 50–75%
Grade 4 – displacement >75%

- Associated with spondylolysis – fracture of the pars interarticularis ("scotty dog" appearance in oblique views)
- Widened anteroposterior diameter of the spinal canal
- Reactive marrow changes
- Endplate sclerosis
- Facet degenerative changes

MANAGEMENT

Immobilization/symptomatic treatment/surgery.

Brachial Plexus Injury with Traumatic Pseudomeningocele

Avulsion injuries of the brachial plexus result in contusion/transection of a nerve root, most commonly at its attachment to the spinal cord. This stretching of the nerve root beyond its maximal capacity leads to tearing of its arachnoid and dural sheaths. This allows leakage of CSF, both along the course of the torn nerve root and along the epidural space.

CLINICAL

History of old trauma, pain, and loss of sensation in the upper limb.

IMAGING

- CSF intensity lesions along the course of exiting nerve roots
- T2/STIR hyperintense perineural edema, involving roots, trunks, and cord of involved brachial plexus
- Non-visualization of normal, isointense nerve roots
- Edema and tear of adjacent paraspinal muscles
- CT myelography reveals nerve root avulsion with bulbous CSF, containing outpouchings in the neural foramina, extending both intra- and extraspinally

DDs

- Post-operative pseudomeningocele

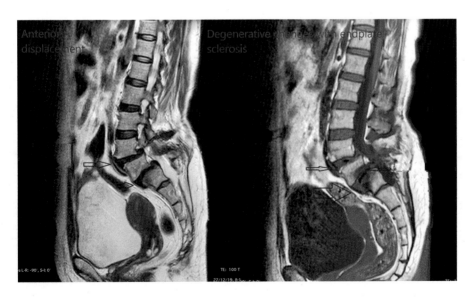

Figure 12.7 Imaging findings of spondylolisthesis.

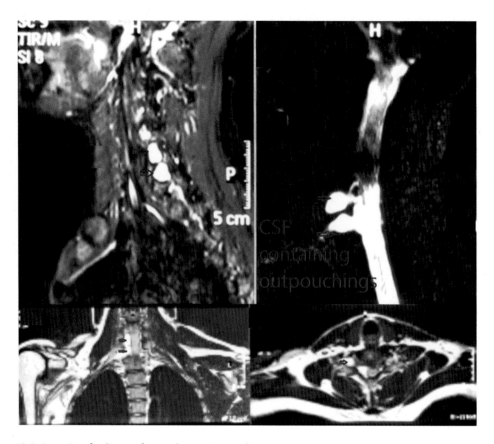

Figure 12.8 Imaging findings of pseudomeningoceles.

MANAGEMENT

Conservative.

Spinal Schwannoma (Neurinoma/Neurilemmoma)

Slow-growing, intradural extramedullary, peripheral nerve sheath tumor can be seen in association with neurofibromatosis (NF2) and schwannomatosis.

CLINICAL

Progressive myelopathy, radiculopathy – weakness and sensory deficit, back pain, paresthesias.

IMAGING

- CT
  - Neural foramina enlargement with the lesion, which may protrude through neural foramina, forming a dumbbell-shaped lesion.

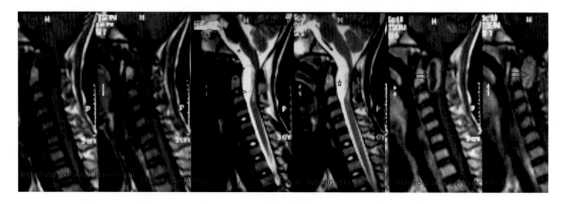

Figure 12.9 Imaging findings of spinal schwannoma.

- Remodeling with scalloping of the posterior vertebral body in large lesions.
- Myelography
  - Spinal cord is deviated contralateral to the mass.
  - Meniscus sign – intradural lesion is demarcated by the sharp meniscus of contrast.
- MRI
  - Heterogeneously isointense on T1W, hyperintense on T2W with intense post-contrast enhancement. Few interspersed hyperintense hemorrhagic foci and cystic areas.

DDs

- Meningioma – homogeneous
- Neurofibroma
- Metastases

MANAGEMENT

Surgery.

Dural Ectasia

Refers to greater-than-normal volume of CSF in thecal sac, and is associated with Marfan's syndrome, neurofibromatosis 1, ankylosing spondylitis, trauma, etc. It results in failed spinal anesthesia.

CLINICAL

Low backache, sphincter dysfunction, muscle weakness.

IMAGING

- Lobulated CSF density, T1 hypointense and T2 hyperintense
- Widening of dural sac
- Vertebral body scalloping
- Herniation of nerve root sleeves

DDs

Tarlov cyst.

Spinal Dural AVF (Arteriovenous Fistula)

Acquired lesions with direct communication between the dural branch of the radicular artery and vein, usually particularly common in male adults after the fifth decade.

CLINICAL

Backache, leg pain with progressive myelopathy.

IMAGING

MRI:

- Serpiginous flow voids in the dorsal subarachnoid space

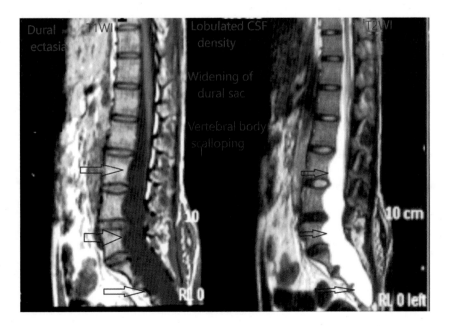

Figure 12.10 Imaging findings of dural ectasia.

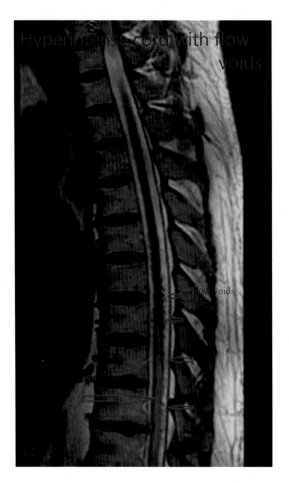

Figure 12.11 Spinal dural AVF.

- Cord expansion
- Intramedullary T1 hypointense and T2 hyperintense signal, contiguous for multiple segments
- Heterogeneous intramedullary enhancement, with enhancing serpiginous vessels
- Myelogram – serpentine filling defects

Angiography:

- Delineates the type and location of fistula and arterial feeders

DDs

- Spinal AVMs – acute presentation with hemorrhage
- CSF flow artifacts – normal cord
- Spinal neoplasms

MANAGEMENT

Endovascular/surgical occlusion.

ANCILLARY

Venous thrombosis may result in subacute necrotizing myelopathy or Foix-Alajouanine syndrome.

Ankylosing Spondylitis (AS)

Chronic, inflammatory, seronegative spondyloarthropathy, HLA-B27 positive, which primarily affects the axial skeleton of young males, 15–35 years old. It may also be associated with abnormalities like inflammatory bowel disease, aortitis, and pulmonary fibrosis.

CLINICAL

Backache and stiffness, especially in the morning.

IMAGING

Sacroiliac Joint

- Bilateral and symmetrical erosions

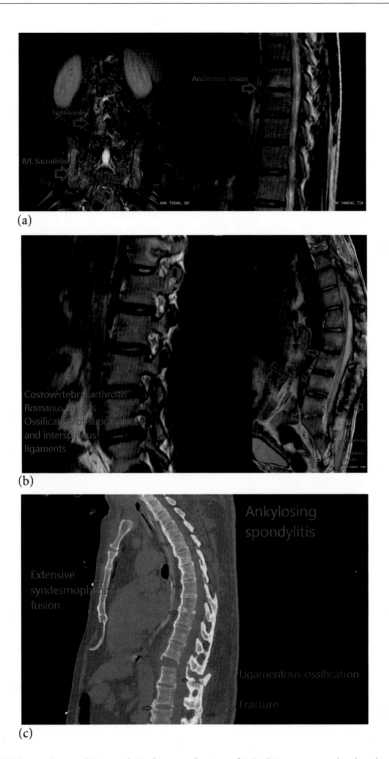

(a)

(b)

(c)

Figure 12.12 (a) Bilateral sacroiliitis and Andersson lesion of AS, (b) costovertebral arthrosis and Romanus lesion, (c) CT findings of AS.

- Joint space widening
- Progressive fusion of sacroiliac joint with ankylosis; subchondral loss is initially on the iliac side of the cartilage complex

Spine

- Squaring of the anterior vertebral margin, with bone erosions at the corners of the vertebral bodies with sclerotic repair (*Romanus lesion with "shiny corner" sign*).
- *Andersson lesions* – inflammatory lesions at the junction of the intervertebral disc and the vertebral endplate, resulting in interbody ankylosis (hyperintense on STIR).
- Syndesmophytes – thin, vertically oriented bony spurs that form an osseous bridge between two adjacent vertebrae, eventually resulting in peripheral spinal ankylosis.
- "*Dagger*" sign – osseous vertical stripe created by fusion of the spinous processes on the frontal projection.
- "*Bamboo spine*" – multilevel spinal fusion with syndesmophytes.
- "*Trolley-track*" *appearance* – three parallel lines of calcification on the anteroposterior projection represents the calcified supraspinous and interspinous ligaments as a central calcific line, with the fused apophyseal joints as peripheral calcifications.
- Prone to fractures through syndesmophytes or vertebral bodies
- Aseptic spondylodiscitis – endplate erosions, sclerosis, and disc calcifications, with sparing of disc space.

MRI:
   Active disease is characterized by:

- Inflammation with subchondral bone marrow edema – hypointense on T1W, hyperintense on STIR/ T2WI, and contrast enhancement
- CEMRI – differentiates enhancing synovium from the hypointense joint effusion
- Chronic disease – T1 hyperintense fatty marrow degeneration

Chronic disease includes subchondral sclerosis, joint space narrowing, bone bridging, and ankylosis, and is low SI on T1 and T2WI.

DDs

- Psoriatic and Reiter's syndrome arthritis involve unilateral sacroiliac joint, or, if both are involved, the sclerotic changes are markedly asymmetrical.
- Rheumatoid arthritis affects synovial membrane, in comparison with AS, which mainly involves entheses (ligamentous and tendinous insertion). Moreover, hands are spared in AS.
- Diffuse idiopathic skeletal hyperostosis (DISH) –thick, flowing pattern of ossification due to bone formation in the anterior longitudinal ligament. Sacroiliac joints are not involved.
- Degenerative bone disease in spondylosis deformans has horizontally oriented osteophytes.
- Osteitis condensans ilii – triangular-shaped hypointense area along the anterior and middle third of the ilium, adjacent to the sacroiliac joints, usually seen in multiparous women, especially during pregnancy.

MANAGEMENT

NSAIDs and intensive physical therapy.

Hangman's Fracture (Traumatic Spondylolisthesis of Axis)

Pars interarticularis fracture of C2 (axis) bilaterally, with distraction and hyperextension as its mechanism. Usually seen in persons who undergo judicial hanging.

CLINICAL

Acute neck pain with a history of trauma. Neurological deficits are less common.

IMAGING

- Fracture of the pedicle of the axis (C2)
- Subluxation of C2 over C3
- Intact odontoid process
- A typical fracture may extend through the vertebral body, and foramen transversarium, and affect vertebral artery

DDs

Chronic spondylolisthesis of axis.

MANAGEMENT

- Collar
- Surgery

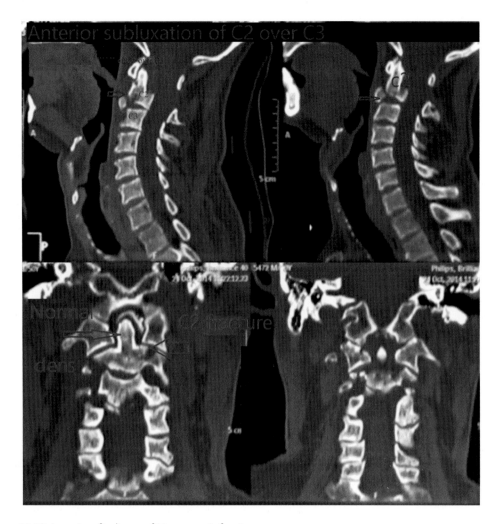

Figure 12.13 Imaging findings of Hangman's fracture.

Vertebral Metastasis with Cord Compression

Secondary involvement of the spine *via* hematogenous dissemination and must be considered as a differential in any osseous lesion in adult patients. The lesions can be lytic/blastic/mixed. The lower thoracic and lumbar spine are the most frequently affected sites.

CLINICAL

Asymptomatic/bone pain, pathological fracture, or cord compression, and eventual neurologic deficits.

IMAGING AND DDs

- PET scan with fluoro-2-deoxy-D-glucose (FDG-PET) – increased glucose metabolism of malignant cells in the bone marrow

- CT myelography – thickened nerve roots and subarachnoid masses, leading to subarachnoid space blockage
- Metastatic lesions show heterogeneous enhancement on CE-MRI, hyperintensity on STIR (fat suppression technique), and restriction on DWI
- Whole-body MRI is mandatory to rule out multiple lesions

OTHER DIFFERENTIALS

- Discitis-osteomyelitis – endplate erosions with abnormal marrow signal and enhancement
  - Intradiscal fluid with patchy enhancement
- Osseous metastases – do not cross the disc space from one vertebral body to the next

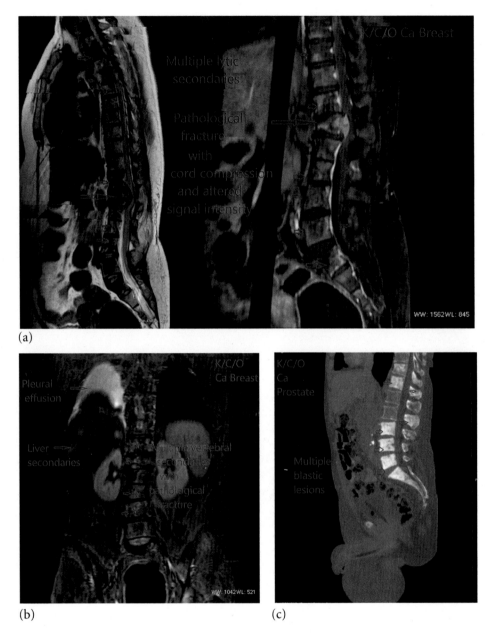

Figure 12.14 (a and b) Multiple secondaries in a k/c/o Ca breast, (c) blastic metastasis in a k/c/o Ca prostate.

ANCILLARY

A lesion that is centered in a vertebral body and extends into the posterior elements is more likely to be malignant than benign.

"Missing pedicle" sign – best visualized on anteroposterior (AP) radiographs. Metastasis tends to involve the posterior vertebral body and pedicle.

Tarlov Cyst (Perineural Cyst)

Benign cysts arising from exiting nerve roots, more commonly in females in the lower lumbar/sacral region.

CLINICAL

Asymptomatic/pressure symptoms (if giant).

IMAGING
CT:

- CSF density lesions
- Bone scalloping

MRI:

- Hypointense on T1W, hyperintense on T2W non-enhancing root sleeve cyst

Myelography:

- Fills with contrast

DDs

- Adnexal cystic lesion
- Other meningeal cysts

MANAGEMENT
Guided aspiration/fibrin injection.

Myxopapillary Ependymoma

Intradural, extramedullary, slow-growing tumor, frequently encountered in the lumbosacral region (conus medullaris/filum terminale), particularly in adult males.

CLINICAL
Backache, muscle weakness, sphincter dysfunction.

IMAGING

- CT – expansion of spinal canal with vertebral body scalloping.
- MRI – well-delineated, lobulated lesion, hypo- to isointense on T1, hyperintense on T2WI/STIR, with variable enhancement. Mucin content may result in high T1 SI and low T2 SI, due to interspersed hemorrhagic areas.

DDs

- Schwannoma
- Astrocytoma
- Paraganglioma

MANAGEMENT
Surgery.

Primary Lymphoma of Spine

Rare tumor.

Table 12.3 Imaging Findings and Differentials of Osteoblastic, Osteolytic, and Mixed Metastases

	Osteoblastic Metastasis	Osteolytic Metastasis	Mixed Lytic-Blastic Metastasis
Common primary	Prostate, osteosarcoma, bronchial carcinoid	Renal cell carcinoma, malignant melanoma, multiple myeloma, lung cancer	Breast carcinoma, lymphoma, urothelial carcinoma
CT	Hyperdense with irregular margins; may extend beyond the vertebrae into the posterior cortex	Soft tissue density lesion with irregular margins. Cortical breach is common, involving the epidural space and reducing canal diameter	Mixed-density appearance
MRI	Hypointense on both T1W and T2W, without any enhancement	Hypointense on T1W and hyperintense on T2W, with avid enhancement	Iso- to hypointense on T1W and iso- to hyperintense on T2W with heterogeneous enhancement
DDs	Bone islands (enostosis), osteoid osteoma, osteoblastoma, post-radio-/chemotherapy	Atypical hemangioma, aneurysmal bone cyst, infectious spondylitis	Osteoid osteoma, osteoblastoma

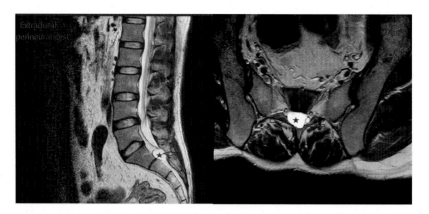

Figure 12.15 Imaging findings of Tarlov cyst.

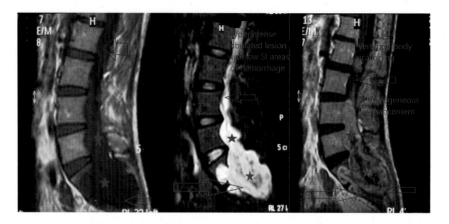

Figure 12.16 Imaging findings of myxopapillary ependymoma.

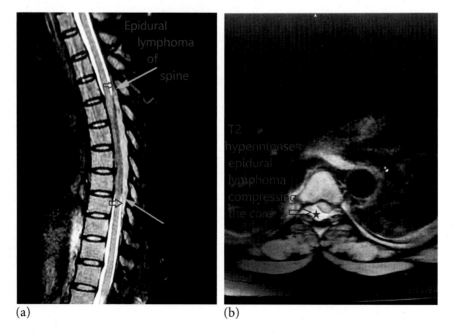

(a)   (b)

Figure 12.17 (a and b) Imaging findings of spinal lymphoma.

CLINICAL

Backache, lower limb weakness, bladder dysfunction.

IMAGING

MRI:

- Isointense on T1WI, hyperintense on T2WI, and homogeneous contrast enhancement
- Cord compression
- Ipsilateral foraminal extension may be seen
- Altered marrow signal
- Associated lymphadenopathy

DDs

- Spinal epidural hematoma – blood products of varying SI
- Epidural abscess – peripheral enhancement
- Epidural metastases

MANAGEMENT

Surgery with radiotherapy.

SUGGESTED READING

Adam, A. *Grainger & Allison's Diagnostic Radiology: A Textbook of Medical Imaging*. Churchill Livingstone; 2008.

Nadgir, R, Yousem, DM. *Neuroradiology: The Requisites*. 4th ed. Philadelphia: Elsevier; 2017.

Osborn, AG, Salzman, KL, Jhaveri, MD, Barkovich, AJ. *Diagnostic Imaging: Brain*. Elsevier Health Sciences; 2015.

Watson, N, Watson, NA. *Jones H. Chapman & Nakielny's Guide to Radiological Procedures*. Elsevier; 2018.

13

Orbit

BOUNDARIES OF THE ORBIT

- The roof constitutes the floor of the frontal sinus and is formed anteriorly by the frontal bone and posteriorly by the lesser wing of the sphenoid bone.
- The medial wall divides the orbit from the ethmoid cells, and is formed by parts of the maxilla, frontal, ethmoid, lacrimal and sphenoid bones. This thin wall (lamina papyracea) is prone to injury.
- The lateral wall is the thickest, separating the orbit from the temporal fossa anteriorly and from the middle cranial fossa posteriorly. It is formed by the greater wing of the sphenoid and the frontal process of the zygomatic bone.
- The floor of the orbit is also thin and prone to blow-out fracture. It contains a passage for the infraorbital nerve and is made up of the zygomatic, maxillary, and palatine bones.

MAJOR APERTURES

- The optic nerve and ophthalmic artery transmit *via* the *optic canal/foramen*, which lies at the orbital apex, through which the orbit communicates with the intracranial cavity posteriorly.
- The *superior orbital fissure (SOF)* is a passage between the orbital apex and the cavernous sinus, and contains the superior ophthalmic vein, the 3rd and 4th cranial nerves, the ophthalmic division of the trigeminal nerve, and the 6th cranial nerve.
- The *inferior orbital fissure*, present between the floor and the lateral wall of the orbit, contains the inferior ophthalmic vein, the infraorbital artery, and the infraorbital nerve (a branch of the maxillary division of trigeminal nerve). The infraorbital foramen crosses the floor of the orbit and carries the infraorbital artery, vein, and nerve from the inferior orbital fissure.

Major anatomical components include the globe, the optic nerve sheath complex, and the conal-intraconal and extraconal areas. The orbital septum is the anterior reflection of its periosteum, and separates the preseptal and post-septal spaces. The post-septal space is further subdivided into intra- and extraconal space by the muscle cone.

GLOBE (OCULAR SPACE)

- The anterior chamber lies between the cornea anteriorly and the lens and iris posteriorly. Pathologies include globe rupture, anterior hyphema (hemorrhage), keratitis, periorbital cellulitis, and cataract.
- The posterior chamber lies behind the iris, with uveitis, glaucoma and ciliary melanoma as the main pathologies.
- The vitreous body lies behind the lens with primary hyperplastic primitive vitreous (PHPV) rupture, hemorrhage, and cytomegalovirus infection as primary pathologies of the region.
- The retina is the innermost lining of the globe and forms part of the optic pathway. Diseases involving this layer include RD (retinal detachment), retinoblastoma, and hemangioblastoma (in association with VHL).
- The choroid, the most vascular structure in the eye, is a part of the uvea, ciliary body, and the iris. Its pathologies include melanoma, metastasis, and detachment.

- The sclera is the outermost layer of the globe, with scleritis, pseudotumor, and infection as the main diseases of this layer.

ORBIT AND OPTIC NERVE SHEATH COMPLEX

The optic nerve sheath complex is formed by the optic nerve and the dural and leptomeningeal coverings. The lesions involving this region include optic neuritis, multiple sclerosis, neuromyelitis optica (Devic's disease), optic nerve glioma, and meningioma.

CONAL-INTRACONAL AREA

The extraocular muscles (EOMs) – the four recti, two obliques, and the levator palpebrae superioris – divide the retro-orbital space into intra- and extraconal spaces. The annulus of Zinn, a fibrous tendon ring, surrounds the optic nerve at the orbital apex and inserts into the globe; it is a common origin for the four recti. Associated lesions include thyroid ophthalmopathy (Graves' disease), and inflammatory pseudotumor.

EXTRACONAL AREA

Lesions in this area include periorbital abscess, orbital and periorbital cellulitis, and sphenoid wing lesions, resulting in proptosis.

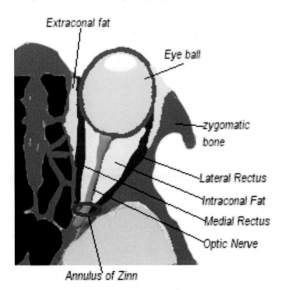

Figure 13.1 Orbital anatomy.

ORBITAL APPENDAGES

- Lacrimal gland – common lesions include inflammation (Sjögren's syndrome, tuberculosis, etc.), dacryocystocele, lymphoma, pleomorphic adenoma, and adenoid cystic tumors
- Lacrimal sac
- Lacrimal duct

CASE STUDIES

Graves' Ophthalmopathy

An autoimmune inflammatory process, that affects the extraocular muscles and orbital fat, is particularly frequent in females, and is associated with thyroid dysfunction.

CLINICAL

Proptosis, lid retraction, impaired color vision, and visual field defects not attributable to other eye diseases.

High serum concentrations of free thyroxine, reduced amount of thyroid-stimulating hormone, and a positive thyrotropin-receptor antibody test.

IMAGING

- Bilateral, symmetrical, and fusiform enlargement (>4 mm) of the non-tendinous part of extraocular muscles (inferior rectus > medial rectus > superior rectus).
- Proptosis (axial scan at the level of the lens). Distance from the interzygomatic line to the anterior cornea >21–23 mm. Asymmetry >2 mm between the two orbits.
- Increased orbital fat volume.
- MRI – isointense on T1 and hyperintense on T2WI, with contrast enhancement.
- Compressive optic neuropathy may occur and need decompression.

DDs

- Orbital myositis – also involves tendinous insertions of EOMs
- Inflammatory pseudotumor – involves the tendinous insertion of EOMs, along with other parts
- Orbital lymphoma
- Metastases

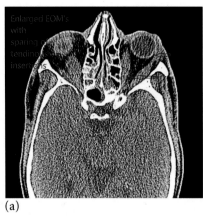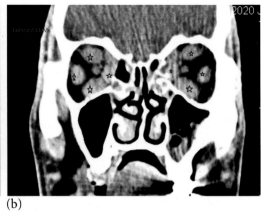

(a)   (b)

Figure 13.2 (a and b) Enlarged extraocular muscles, with sparing of tendinous insertions.

MANAGEMENT

Conservative treatment.

Orbital Pseudotumor

Non-neoplastic, idiopathic inflammatory process of the orbit, usually unilateral, and frequently affects middle-aged individuals.

CLINICAL

Painful exophthalmos, reduced ocular motility, diplopia, ptosis, chemosis, uveal, and scleral thickening.

IMAGING

- CT – focal or diffusely enhancing intraorbital (intraconal/extraconal) mass
  - Associated infiltration of the retrobulbar fat, lacrimal gland involvement, edema, bone destruction, and intracranial extension
- MRI – enlargement of the extraocular muscles, with the involvement of their tendinous insertions

- Isointense on T1WI, hypo- (sclerosing variant due to fibrosis) to hyperintense (acute/subacute inflammatory nature) on T2WI, with moderate to marked diffuse post-contrast enhancement
- DWI – restricted diffusion
  - Delineates intracranial extension *via* superior or inferior orbital fissure

DDs

- Graves' ophthalmopathy – painless and spares the tendinous insertions
- Orbital lymphoma – slowly progressive, bilateral, and does not respond to corticosteroid treatment
- Orbital cellulitis – subperiosteal abscess and paranasal sinus involvement
- Tolosa-Hunt syndrome, orbital sarcoidosis, metastasis, and rhabdomyosarcoma

MANAGEMENT

- Systemic corticosteroid therapy – dramatic improvement within 24 to 48 hours

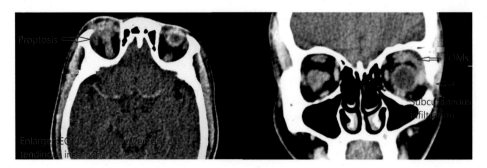

Figure 13.3 Enlarged extraocular muscles, with involvement of tendinous insertions.

- Low-dose radiation

Optic Neuritis

Inflammation of the optic nerve (retrobulbar intra-orbital segment). More common in young females.

CLINICAL

Painful, unilateral subacute visual loss.

IMAGING

- MRI – optic nerve appears enlarged/swollen in acute cases, with a high T2/ STIR signal which persists chronically, even when the optic nerve atrophies
- Fat-suppressed T1 coronal image depicts contrast enhancement

DDs

- Toxic/nutritional optic neuropathy – bilateral, symmetrical, and painless
- Ischemic optic neuropathy
- Optic perineuritis – enhancement around the optic nerve ("tram track"/"doughnut" sign)

MANAGEMENT

Self-limiting, with recovery of vision commencing within a few weeks of symptom onset.
    Intravenous steroids may hasten recovery.

ANCILLARY

Associated with:

- Multiple sclerosis – unilateral

- Acute disseminated encephalomyelitis (ADEM) – usually bilateral and occurs after vaccination or viral infection

Tolosa-Hunt Syndrome

Idiopathic, inflammatory granulomatous disease, involving the orbital apex and the cavernous sinus. It is a clinical diagnosis of exclusion, with the pain being relieved within three days of steroid therapy.

CLINICAL

Recurrent, unilateral, painful ophthalmoplegia, with neuropathy involving the 3rd, 4th, and 6th cranial nerves.

IMAGING

- CT – asymmetrical enlargement of the ipsilateral cavernous sinus
- MRI – isointense on T1WI and T2WI, with abnormal enlargement and enhancement of the cavernous sinus, extending into the orbital apex through the superior orbital fissure
- Angiography – focal narrowing of the cavernous ICA and the superior ophthalmic vein

DDs

- Ophthalmoplegic migraine (oculomotor palsy) – enhancement of cisternal segment of 3rd cranial nerve, with no involvement of the cavernous sinus
- Miller-Fisher syndrome – painless, bilateral ophthalmoplegia and ataxia
- Caroticocavernous fistula
- Metastases, lymphoma, sarcoidosis

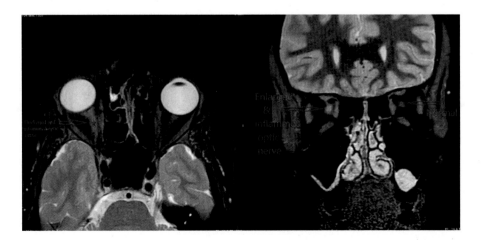

Figure 13.4 Imaging findings of optic neuritis.

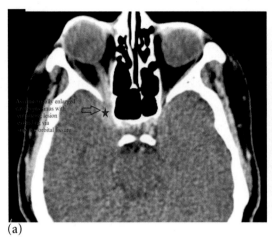
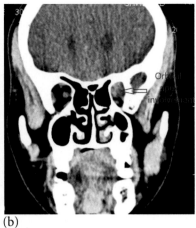

(a) (b)

Figure 13.5 (a and b) Imaging findings of Tolosa-Hunt syndrome.

Retinoblastoma

The most common type of intraocular tumors in children.

PNETs associated with hereditary retinoblastoma → trilateral/quadrilateral retinoblastoma (pineal/suprasellar region).

CLINICAL

Leukocoria (white pupil reflection), squint.

IMAGING

Three patterns of growth – endophytic, exophytic, or mixed.

- CT – heterogeneously hyperdense mass, with areas of necrosis and calcifications
- CECT – moderately enhancing
- MRI – intermediate signal intensity on T1WI, and hypointense on T2WI, with heterogeneous post-contrast enhancement
  - Delineates optic nerve involvement, ocular, and intracranial extension
- DWI – restricted diffusion

DDs

- Non-neoplastic lesions that also cause leukocoria and Coats disease, Toxocara granulomatosis, retinopathy of prematurity, and retinal astrocytic hamartoma

MANAGEMENT

Surgery with external-beam radiation therapy/laser photocoagulation.

Optic Nerve Glioma

Usually low grade, common in children, where it occurs in association with neurofibromatosis type 1 (NF1). Rare but aggressive in adults, without any association with NF1.

CLINICAL

Reduced vision, proptosis, symptoms of raised ICP, focal neurological deficits.

IMAGING

- CT – enlarged optic nerve with fusiform or exophytic lesion, exhibiting variable enhancement
- MRI – large tumors are typically heterogeneous, with cystic and solid components; iso- to hypointense on T1WI and hyperintense on T2WI, with variable enhancement

DDs

As per classification:

- Stage 1: Optic nerves only (DDs – meningioma with calcifications and "tram track" appearance, hemangioma, lymphoma, and metastases)
- Stage 2: Chiasm ± optic nerve involvement (DDs – germinoma, sarcoidosis)
- Stage 3: Hypothalamic involvement (DDs – pituitary adenoma, craniopharyngioma, malignant astrocytoma)

MANAGEMENT

Surgery, depending on the stage of the lesion.

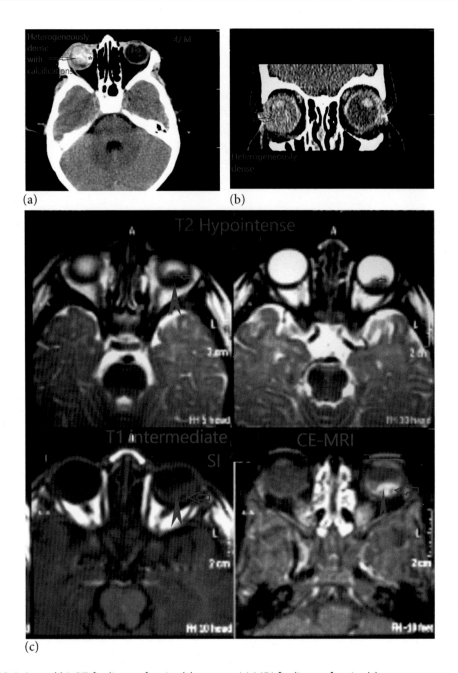

Figure 13.6 (a and b) CT findings of retinoblastoma, (c) MRI findings of retinoblastoma.

Choroidal Melanoma (Uveal Melanoma)

Most frequent cause of intraocular tumors in adults.

CLINICAL

Visual field defects, visual loss, pain, and photopsia (perceived flashes of light).

IMAGING

- CT – hyperdense, elevated, mushroom-shaped lesion, with diffuse, moderate enhancement
- MR – hyperintense on T1WI (owing to paramagnetic effects of melanin) and hypointense on T2WI, showing diffuse moderate enhancement

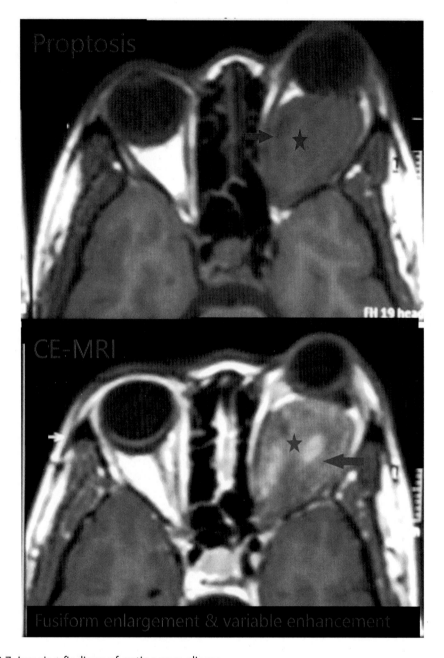

Figure 13.7 Imaging findings of optic nerve glioma.

DDs

- Choroidal metastases (from lung, breast, hypervascular, and hematologic malignancies) – bilateral, multiple, and hyperintense on T2WI.
- Choroidal hemangioma – hypointense on T1WI and hyperintense on T2WI.
- Vitreous hemorrhage – hyperintense on T1WI and hypointense on T2WI (intracellular methemoglobin), but do not show enhancement.
- Melanocytic nevi (orbital melanocytoma) – difficult to differentiate on imaging.
- Retinoblastoma – involves younger population, and shows calcifications. Hypointense on T1WI, hyperintense on T2WI and enhances heterogeneously.

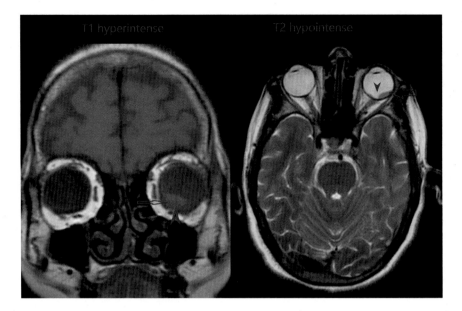

Figure 13.8 Imaging findings of choroidal melanoma.

MANAGEMENT

Transpupillary thermotherapy, plaque brachy-therapy, or external-beam radiation therapy for smaller melanomas and surgical enucleation for the larger ones.

Orbital Blow-Out Fracture

Fracture due to blunt trauma with intact orbital rim.

CLINICAL

Enophthalmos, orbital restriction, strabismus, and diplopia, especially on vertical gaze. Entrapment of the inferior rectus muscle results in oculocardiac reflex, especially in the pediatric population, with a triad of bradycardia, nausea, and syncope.

IMAGING

CT:

- Inferior blow-out fracture (floor) – fragments, inferior rectus muscle, and fat herniates into the antrum
- Medial fracture (lamina papyracea), with herniation of fat and medial rectus muscle into ethmoid air cells

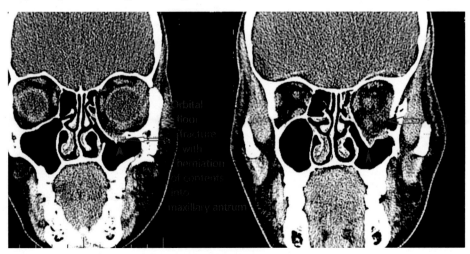

Figure 13.9 Imaging findings of orbital blow-out fracture.

- Orbital roof fracture – CSF leak or herniation of brain tissue or meninges into the orbit
- Soft tissue swelling
- Intramuscular hematoma
- Orbital emphysema

MRI:

- Contraindicated if there is suspicion of a metallic foreign body

MANAGEMENT

- Uncomplicated cases – conservative management
- Surgery – muscle entrapment, fracture area >50% of the orbital floor, and significant enophthalmos

ANCILLARY

Blow-in fractures – superior displacement of the orbital floor.

Cavernous Hemangioma

Most frequent vascular lesions of the orbit in adults; usually, they involve the lateral aspect of the retrobulbar intraconal space, and occur most often in females, but do not involute.

CLINICAL

Slowly progressive, painless proptosis, associated with headache, lid swelling, diplopia, a palpable lump, and recurrent episodes of obscured vision.

IMAGING

- NCCT – well-circumscribed, round or ovoid, homogeneously hyperdense, intraconal lesion

Microcalcifications (phleboliths)
- Expansion of the orbital walls
- May displace adjacent structures but do not invade them
- CECT
- Poor enhancement in the early arterial phase (owing to low-flow arterial supply)
- Filling of the central part of the lesion in the late venous phase
- Delayed wash-out
- MRI – T1 isointense and T2 hyperintense lesion (hypointense capsule on T2), with progressive accumulation of contrast material on late-phase dynamic images and delayed images.
- Conventional angiography with a prolonged injection – delayed contrast material pooling.

DDs

- Intraconal meningioma, schwannoma
- Orbital metastasis
- Orbital lymphoma
- Vascular lesions with early arterial phase enhancement – capillary hemangiomas, hemangiopericytomas. No delayed pooling and wash-out
- High-flow arteriovenous malformations, carotid-cavernous fistulas, and aneurysms

MANAGEMENT

Conservative management. Surgical excision for complicated cases with severe proptosis or optic nerve compression.

ANCILLARY

Capillary hemangiomas are among the most frequent benign orbital tumors of infancy, with fast growth in infancy and spontaneous involution

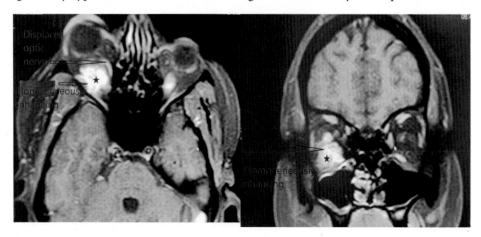

Figure 13.10 Imaging findings of cavernous hemangioma.

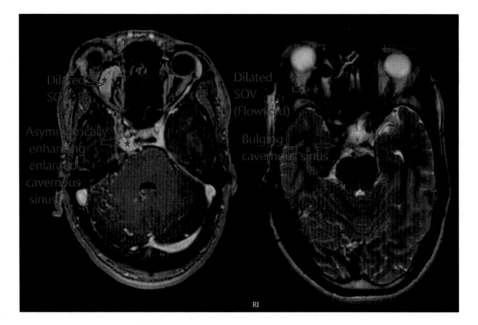

Figure 13.11 Imaging findings of carotid-cavernous fistula.

later in life. Does not present at birth, but almost always develops by six months of age. Management is usually conservative, with excellent prognosis and involution of most tumors by five years of age.

Carotid-Cavernous Fistula

Abnormal communication between the cavernous sinus and carotid vessels. It can be direct (post-traumatic, usually) or indirect (spontaneous)/high-flow *vs* low-flow.

CLINICAL

Pulsatile proptosis, chemosis, visual deficits, signs of raised ICP.

IMAGING

CT/MRI:

- Exophthalmos with orbital congestion
- Enlarged extraocular muscles
- Dilated superior ophthalmic vein (SOV) >4 mm/flow voids on MRI
- Bulging, asymmetrically enhancing cavernous sinus
- Angiography

- Determination of type and localization of fistulous connection between the carotid artery and the cavernous sinus
- Retrograde filling of superior ophthalmic vein

DDs

- Tolosa-Hunt syndrome
- Vascular malformations

MANAGEMENT

Endovascular treatment.

SUGGESTED READING

Grech, R, Cornish, KS, Galvin, PL, Grech, S, Looby, S, O'Hare, A, Mizzi, A, Thornton, J, Brennan, P. Imaging of adult ocular and orbital pathology—A pictorial review. *Journal of Radiology Case Reports* 2014;8(2):1–29.

Hande, PC, Talwar, I. Multimodality imaging of the orbit. *Indian Journal of Radiology & Imaging* 2012;22(3):227–239.

Osborn, AG, Salzman, KL, Jhaveri, MD, Barkovich, AJ. *Diagnostic Imaging: Brain.* Elsevier Health Sciences; 2015.

14

Neck

The neck is divided into anterior and posterior triangles by the sternocleidomastoid muscle. The hyoid bone divides the anterior triangle into the suprahyoid and the infrahyoid neck regions.

NECK SPACES OF SUPRA- AND INFRAHYOID REGION AND FASCIAL LAYERS

Fascial layers:

- Superficial cervical fascia (subcutaneous fat, veins, nerves, lymphatics, platysma, and facial muscles)
- Deep cervical fascia (DCF)
  - Superficial layer (investing layer)
  - Middle layer (visceral/pretracheal)
  - Deep layer (prevertebral)

VISCERAL SPACE

Contents: Naso- and oropharynx, mucosa, lymphoid tissue of Waldeyer's ring (adenoids, tonsils), minor salivary glands, hypopharynx, larynx, thyroid. trachea, parathyroid, and cervical esophagus.

RETROPHARYNGEAL SPACE (RPS)

The RPS is confined anteriorly by the visceral fascia and posteriorly by the prevertebral fascia. A thin alar fascia layer divides the RPS into anterior and posterior compartments. The posterior compartment (danger space) continues from the skull base to the diaphragm. It is a channel for the cranial and cervical infection and tumors to extend into the mediastinum.

Contents: Fat (predominantly) and retropharyngeal lymph nodes (RPLN, nodes of Rouviere).

PREVERTEBRAL SPACE (PVS)

The PVS is enclosed by the prevertebral fascia and lies posteriorly to the retropharyngeal space.

Contents: Prevertebral muscles (longus colli capitis), vertebral body, cervical disk, spinal canal, vertebral artery, and phrenic nerve.

PERIVERTEBRAL SPACE

It completely encircles the vertebral body, including the pre- and paravertebral muscles.

PARAPHARYNGEAL SPACE (PPS)

It is also known as the prestyloid parapharyngeal space, lies next to the pharynx and extends from the skull base to the hyoid bone.

Contents: Fat, vascular structures, small branches of the 5th cranial nerve, lymph nodes, and ectopic rests of the minor salivary gland tissue.

PHARYNGEAL MUCOSAL SPACE (PMS)

Contents: Pharynx, lymph nodes, adenoids, and minor salivary glands.

CAROTID SPACE (CS)/POST-STYLOID PPS, CAROTID SHEATH

It is formed by all three layers of deep fascia.

Contents: Internal carotid artery, internal jugular vein, cranial nerves IX to XII, sympathetic chain, and lymph nodes.

MASTICATOR SPACE (MS)

Contents: Muscles of mastication (medial and lateral pterygoid, masseter, and temporalis), ramus of the mandible, and the mandibular division of the trigeminal nerve.

PAROTID SPACE

It contains the parotid gland and is demarcated into the superficial and deep lobes by the facial nerve, which is located just lateral to the retromandibular vein.

Contents: Gland parenchyma, facial nerve, retromandibular vein, external carotid artery, and intraparotid lymph nodes.

BUCCAL SPACE

Contents: Adipose tissue, minor salivary gland tissue, parotid duct, lymph nodes, facial vein, facial and buccal artery, and buccal branch of the 5th and 7th cranial nerves.

SUBLINGUAL SPACE (SLS)/FLOOR OF MOUTH

Space located below the tongue is enclosed by the mylohyoid muscle and the hyoid bone.

Contents: Hypoglossal nerve, the lingual nerve, lingual artery and vein, sublingual gland and ducts, the deep component of the submandibular gland and duct, and lymph nodes.

SUBMANDIBULAR SPACE (SMS)

It is located below the mandible, inferior to the mylohyoid muscle, with the hyoid bone as its inferior margin. Its posterior part communicates directly with the posterior side of the SLS.

Contents: Anterior belly of the digastric muscle, superficial portion of the submandibular gland, facial artery and vein, fat, inferior loop of the hypoglossal nerve, submandibular and submental lymph nodes.

VASCULAR STRUCTURES OF THE NECK

The subclavian artery (SCA) is the main vessel supplying the neck, brain, and upper limb. The right SCA arises from the inominate artery

(brachiocephalic trunk) and the left SCA arises from the arch of the aorta.

The branches of the SCA include:

- The vertebral artery
- The internal thoracic artery
- The thyro-cervical artery
  - The inferior thyroid
  - The subscapular
  - The transverse cervical
- The costocervical artery
  - The superior intercostal
  - The deep cervical
- The dorsal scapular artery

At C3–5 levels, the common carotid artery bifurcates into the external and internal carotid arteries.

Branches of the External Carotid Artery

- The superior thyroid artery
- The ascending pharyngeal artery
- The lingual artery
- The facial artery
- The occipital artery
- The posterior auricular artery
- The superficial temporal artery (characteristic hairpin turn on an angiogram, where it crosses the zygomatic arch)
- The internal maxillary artery

The subclavian vein, brachiocephalic vein, and internal jugular vein receive the blood from the neck.

SALIVARY GLANDS

The parotid gland, the largest salivary gland, is separated, by the retromandibular or facial vein, into the larger superficial and smaller deep lobes. It is situated posterior to the mandibular ramus and drains *via* Stenson's duct, which opens into the oral cavity at the ipsilateral second maxillary molar. The gland parenchyma is nearly isodense/isointense to fat on computed tomography/magnetic resonance imaging (CT/MR) images. It normally has many intraparenchymal and surrounding lymph nodes.

The submandibular gland, the second-largest salivary gland, is situated on the floor of the mouth, proximate to the posterior body of mandible along the free edge of the mylohyoid muscle. The lingual nerve and submandibular ganglion lie superficial to the submandibular gland, whereas the hypoglossal nerve lies deep to it. It drains *via* Wharton's duct into the papilla in the sublingual region.

The sublingual gland is the smallest major salivary gland and lies submucosally adjacent to the anterior mandible in a parasymphyseal location. Wharton's duct and the lingual nerve separate the sublingual gland from the medial genioglossus muscle. Secretions drain, *via* multiple ducts of Rivinus, directly into the floor of the mouth along sublingual papilla and folds.

LYMPH NODES OF THE NECK

- *Level I* includes all the nodes above the hyoid bone and below the mylohyoid muscle:
  - Level IA represents the submental nodes, between the anterior bellies of the digastric muscles.
  - Level IB represents the submandibular nodes, around the submandibular gland.
- *Level II* (upper jugular) nodes extend from the skull base to the level of the lower body of the hyoid bone.
  - Level IIA nodes lie anterior, lateral, medial, and posterior to the internal jugular vein (IJV), and the posterior ones are inseparable from the IJV.
  - Level II B lies posterior to the IJV and can be separated from it.
- *Level III* (mid-jugular) nodes lie between the hyoid bone and cricoid cartilage.

- *Level IV* (low jugular) nodes lie between the lower margin of the cricoid cartilage arch and the supraclavicular fossa.
- *Level V* includes the posterior triangle or spinal accessory nodes, that lie posterior to the posterior margin of the sternocleidomastoid muscle.
- *Level VI* (visceral) nodes represent the central compartment nodes from the hyoid bone to the suprasternal notch, with the carotid sheaths as the lateral border.
- *Level VII* nodes lie inferior to the suprasternal notch in the upper mediastinum.

All nodes greater than 10 mm in diameter should be evaluated for metastasis, infectious, or inflammatory etiologies.

Infective lymphadenitis exhibits homogeneous enhancement, loss of fatty hilum and adjacent fat stranding in initial stages, followed by suppuration with central liquefactive necrosis and rim enhancement.

Metastatic nodes are usually matted, necrotic, and show extracapsular spread, with infiltration to adjacent fat or muscle.

LARYNX

The larynx continues from the tip of the epiglottis to the cricoid cartilage inferiorly. It is divided into:

- The supraglottis, extending from the superior tip of epiglottis to the transverse plane, through the laryngeal ventricle

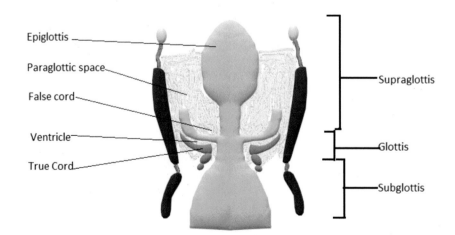

Figure 14.1 Anatomy of larynx.

- The glottis, which extends through the above-mentioned transverse plane to 1 cm inferiorly and includes true vocal cords
- The subglottis, extending from the inferior surface of the true vocal cords to the cricoid cartilage inferiorly

It includes three unpaired cartilages, namely the epiglottis, thyroid, and the cricoid, and the paired arytenoid cartilages.

The epiglottis is the leaf-shaped cartilage in the midline with a free margin (attachment for the hyoepiglottic ligament, which is near the base of the tongue) and a fixed portion called the stem (attachment for the thyroepiglottic ligament).

The thyroid cartilage has superior and inferior cornua, articulating to the thyrohyoid ligament and the cricothyroid joint, respectively.

The cricoid is the ring-shaped laryngeal cartilage.

The arytenoid cartilages are paired and sit along the upper margin of the cricoid lamina, forming the cricoarytenoid joints.

Non-ossified cartilages like the epiglottis and the vocal processes of the arytenoids have soft tissue attenuations on CT and intermediate signal intensity (SI) on T1W and T2WI. The thyroid, cricoid, and arytenoids are hyaline cartilages that show progressive ossification with age and have dense peripheral margins with hypodense medullary cavities. On MRI, the ossified cortical margins are hypointense and the fat-filled medullary cavity is hyperintense on T1W and T2WI.

THYROID

The developing thyroid gland is a diverticulum, connected by the thyroglossal duct, ventral to the hyoid, to the tongue base at the foramen cecum. The thyroglossal duct normally involutes. Internal carotid arteries and internal jugular veins lie posterolateral to thyroid lobes, while strap muscles of the neck lie anteriorly. NCCT scans exhibit homogenous high attenuation values (owing to high iodine concentration) in comparison with adjacent muscles. CECT demonstrates avid enhancement, as a result of hypervascularity. On MRI, the thyroid appears hyperintense on T1 and T2WI, with strong homogeneous enhancement.

The thymus and the inferior parathyroid originate from the third pharyngeal pouch. The fourth pharyngeal pouch gives rise to the superior parathyroid glands.

CASE STUDIES

Thyroglossal Duct Cyst (TGDC)

This is a congenital anomaly of the neck, which can occur anywhere between the foramen cecum to the final position of the thyroid in the anterior neck, due to the persistent thyroglossal duct. It may be associated with ectopic thyroid tissue.

CLINICAL

Non-tender, mobile, midline mass that typically moves upward, with protrusion of the tongue and swallowing, owing to its connection at the base of the tongue.

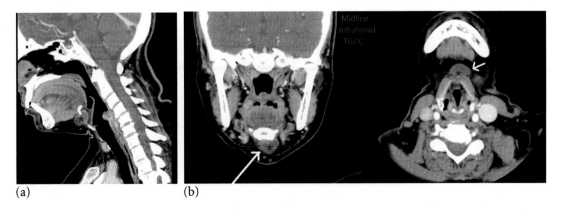

(a)   (b)

Figure 14.2 (a and b) Imaging findings of thyroglossal duct cysts.

IMAGING

- NCCT – midline, thin-walled, smooth, cystic (hypodense) neck mass, embedded in infrahyoid strap muscles and displacing the sternocleidomastoid posterolaterally
- CECT – peripheral rim enhancement
- MRI – intermediate SI on T1W (high SI may be seen if the contents are proteinaceous or hemorrhagic) and hyperintense signal on T2WI

DDs

- Branchial cleft cyst (BCC) – located laterally
- Dermoid cysts – usually hyperechoic/dense, due to hair and sebaceous glands, commonly located at the suprasternal notch and the outer orbit
- Epidermoid cyst – superficial to strap muscles
- Saccular cysts/laryngoceles – congenital dilatation of the saccule of the laryngeal ventricle in the supraglottic region
- Necrotic lymph nodes – usually multiple, with irregular central cystic changes

MANAGEMENT

Sistrunk operation, *en bloc* resection of the cyst, and thyroglossal duct.

ANCILLARY

Cysts located above the level of the thyroid cartilage are usually midline, whereas cysts located below the level of the thyroid cartilage are off midline.

Branchial Cleft Cyst (BCC)

The second BCC is the most common of all BCCs; typically, they occur at the angle of the mandible, displace the submandibular gland anteriorly, the carotid artery and jugular vein medially, and the sternocleidomastoid posteriorly.

CLINICAL

Painless, compressible neck masses in childhood or early adulthood, which may become painful if infected.

IMAGING

- NCCT – unilocular, hypodense, non-enhancing cystic lesion, with an imperceptible wall, in a characteristic location. If infected, it will appear thick-walled, with peripheral enhancement and surrounding inflammatory stranding on CECT.
- MRI – typically, CSF intensity on T1 and T2WI.

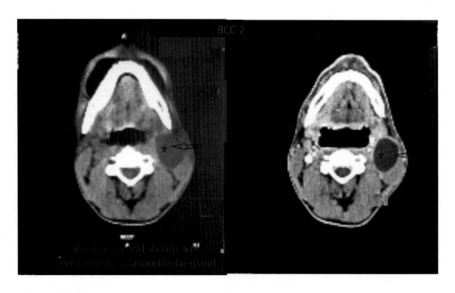

Figure 14.3 Second BCC.

DDs

- Off-midline thyroglossal duct cyst
- Cystic/necrotic lymph node (metastatic due to squamous cell carcinoma/ papillary carcinoma of the thyroid and tuberculosis)
- The dermoid constitutes a mixed-density lesion with fat, fluid, and calcific components, with a "sac of marbles" appearance
- Epidermoid cysts
- Lymphatic malformation
- Cystic vagal schwannoma
- Ranula

MANAGEMENT

Surgical excision.

ANCILLARY

- Spectrum of branchial apparatus anomalies results from incomplete obliteration, proliferation, or migration of one of the four branchial clefts:
  - BC cyst – no internal or external communication
  - BC fistula – has both internal and external communications
  - BC sinus – opens internally (most commonly) or externally, with closed portion ending as a blind pouch

Other Types of Branchial Cleft Cysts

- The first BCC can occur around the external auditory canal (Type I) or in a periparotid

location (Type II), between the EAC and the angle of the mandible.

- The third BCC can occur, either in the upper neck (posterior cervical space) or along the anterior border of the sternocleidomastoid in the lower neck.
- The fourth BCC can occur anywhere from the pyriform sinus apex to the superior thyroid lobe.

Cystic Hygroma (Nuchal Lymphangioma)

Benign congenital abnormalities of the lymphatic system, with the posterior cervical space of the neck being the most common site. Other sites include the submandibular space, axilla, mediastinum, groin, and retroperitoneum.

CLINICAL

Painless neck mass. Infection, trauma, or hemorrhage in the lesion may result in pain, dyspnea, or respiratory compromise.

IMAGING

- CT – non-enhancing, hypodense, multiloculated lesion, with enhancement of septations. The lesion can infiltrate into adjacent fascial planes.
- MRI – T1-hypointense, T2-hyperintense, non-enhancing lesion, with enhancing septa.

DDs

- Occipital encephalocele is usually without septations and in direct continuity with the

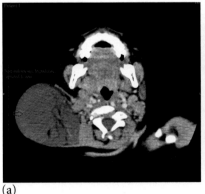 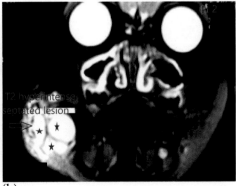

(a)   (b)

Figure 14.4 (a and b) Imaging findings of cystic hygroma.

calvarial defect, through which the brain tissue herniates

- Cervical meningocele

MANAGEMENT

Surgical resection.

Laryngocele

Abnormal dilation of the laryngeal ventricle saccule/appendix. Acquired laryngoceles, such as are caused by coughing, trumpet playing, glassblowing, or tumor obstruction, resulting in elevated laryngeal pressure, and are more common than congenital ones. Secondary laryngoceles may occur when the tumor obstructs the orifice of the laryngeal ventricle and causes laryngocele.

CLINICAL

Asymptomatic. Palpable neck lump, dysphagia, sore throat, or shortness of breath in cases where the lesion becomes enlarged or an infection sets in (pyolaryngocele).

IMAGING

- CT – air-/fluid-filled lesion in the paraglottic space, which is connected with the airways.

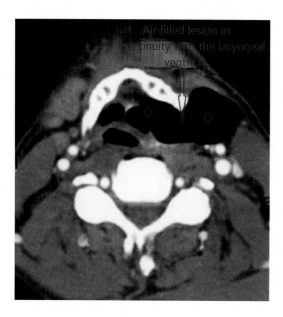

Figure 14.5 Laryngocele.

Rim enhancement and fluid levels may be seen in complicated cases. Search for any tumor obstructing the orifice.

- MRI – T1-hypointense, T2-hyperintense lesion, with absent to minimal peripheral enhancement.

DDs

- Saccular/laryngeal cyst does not show any communication with the laryngeal lumen
- Thyroglossal duct cyst
- Branchial cleft cyst
- Ectasia of internal jugular vein

MANAGEMENT

- Surgical (endoscopic) management for symptomatic lesions. Drainage with antibiotics for pyolaryngoceles, prior to excision. Marsupialization of internal laryngoceles.

ANCILLARY

Laryngoceles can be:

- Internal – confined to larynx in the false vocal fold and the aryepiglottic fold, medial to the thyrohyoid membrane
- External – extend through the thyrohyoid membrane, with dilatation of only the extra laryngeal component
- Mixed – dilatation of saccules on both sides of the thyrohyoid membrane

The laryngeal ventricle lies between the supraglottis and the glottis anatomically. It is a slit-like cavity between the false and the true vocal cords.

Calcific Longus Colli Tendonitis (Retropharyngeal/Acute Calcific Prevertebral Tendonitis)

Inflammatory/granulomatous response to calcium hydroxyapatite crystal deposition of the longus colli muscle, usually seen anterior to the C1–C2 disc space, and in middle-aged females.

CLINICAL

Neck pain, reduced movement of neck, odynophagia. Laboratory tests may reveal leukocytosis, elevated C-reactive protein (CRP), and ESR.

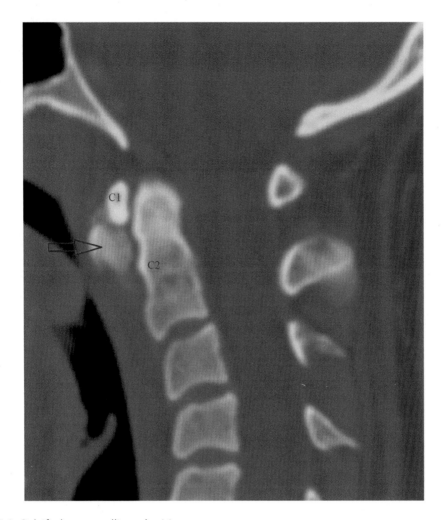

Figure 14.6 Calcific longus colli tendonitis.

IMAGING
NCCT:

- Calcification of longus colli muscle fibers
- Edematous and hypodense muscle
- Edema of adjacent prevertebral soft tissues
- Small non-enhancing retropharyngeal effusions
- Not associated with any adenopathy or bony destruction

MRI:

- Edema and retropharyngeal effusion

DDs

- Trauma – prevertebral bone fragments may simulate muscle calcification
- Retropharyngeal abscess – peripheral enhancement, restricted diffusion, and associated lymphadenopathy
- Tumor – soft tissue component, with contrast enhancement and associated lymphadenopathy
- Infectious spondylodiscitis – associated disc narrowing and inflammatory changes

MANAGEMENT

Self-resolving and requires conservative management, with non-steroidal anti-inflammatory drugs (NSAIDs).

ANCILLARY

The longus colli muscle lies on the anterior surface of the vertebral column, extending from the C1 to

T3 levels. It consists of vertical, superior, and inferior oblique parts; the upper myotendinous junction of the superior oblique part is involved frequently.

Retropharyngeal Abscess (RPA)

Penetrating injury, foreign body, or resulting infection from Gram-positive cocci are the most frequent causes of RP space infections in adults.

In children, upper respiratory tract infection/pharyngitis, due to *Haemophilus influenzae*, spreads to RPS and nodes, resulting in suppuration, which, if not treated, may rupture, leading to RP abscess.

CLINICAL

Children under five years of age and immuno-compromised adults are prone to RPA, and may present with fever, poor feeding, generalized irritability, unilateral neck swelling, palpable lymphadenopathy, and stridor.

IMAGING

- Plain X-ray film (inspiratory image taken in extension) – widening of prevertebral stripe with soft-tissue edema to 7 mm or more at C2, or, at C6, more than 14 mm (children) or more than 22 mm (adults).
- CT – hypodense fluid collection with peripherally enhancing walls in RPS, with moderate to marked mass effect, that displaces the pharynx anteriorly and flattens the prevertebral muscles. The collection may contain gas locules.
- MRI – hypointense T1W, hyperintense T2W SI, with peripheral enhancement on CE-MRI and restricted diffusion on DWI.

COMPLICATIONS

- Anterior extension may compromise airways
- Posterior extension to prevertebral space leads to epidural abscess, discitis
- Lateral extension may involve carotid artery and jugular vein, resulting in hemorrhage, thrombosis, stenosis, or pseudoaneurysm
- Inferiorly, it may extend from the skull base to the mediastinum
- Systemic dissemination may lead to sepsis

DDs

- Suppurative lymph node
- RP edema – lacks enhancing wall and produces less of a mass effect and may be associated with calcification of the longus colli tendon anterior to C1–C2
- Prevertebral abscess – look for vertebral bodies, disc space
- RP cellulitis – phlegmonous thickening
- RP hematoma

MANAGEMENT

Intravenous antibiotics and surgical drainage, when necessary.

Carotid Body Tumor

Neuroendocrine tumor of the carotid body (a chemoreceptor at the carotid bifurcation), these glomus tumors of head, neck, or paragangliomas are rare, highly vascular tumors, affecting females predominantly.

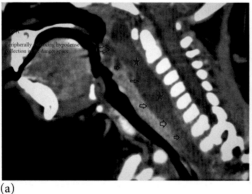
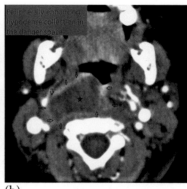

(a)   (b)

Figure 14.7 (a and b) Imaging findings of RPA.

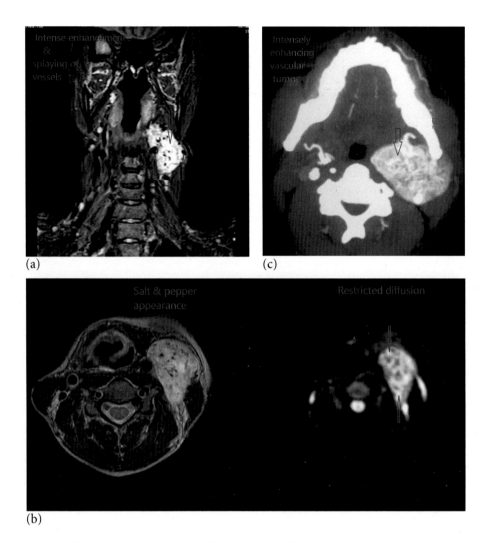

Figure 14.8 (a and b) MRI findings of carotid body tumor, (c) CT findings of carotid body tumor.

CLINICAL

Mobile, non-tender, slow-growing, lateral neck masses with associated hoarseness, dysphagia (tracheal or esophageal compression), vertigo, and cranial nerve palsies.

IMAGING

- CECT – intensely enhancing heterogeneous mass (due to areas of hemorrhage or necrosis), that splays the internal and external carotid artery at the carotid bifurcation.
- MRI – "salt and pepper" appearance, due to multiple flow voids ("pepper") and hyperintensity due to slow-flow/hemorrhage/intrinsic tumor neovascularity ("salt"). The lesion is isointense on T1W and hyperintense on T2W, with intense enhancement.
- DWI – show restriction.
- Angiography – splaying of carotid vessels (Lyre sign), along with strong capillary blush, intense neovascularity, and arteriovenous shunting.

DDs

- Vagal schwannomas – heterogeneously enhancing lesions displacing both the vessels together, instead of splaying them
- Lymph nodes or nodal metastasis

MANAGEMENT

Surgical removal with or without preoperative embolization, to help reduce blood loss.

ANCILLARY

Other locations of glomus tumors include:

- Jugular bulb (glomus jugulare)
- Middle ear cavity (glomus tympanicum)
- Vagus nerve (glomus vagale)

Laryngeal Carcinoma

The most frequent primary malignant tumor of the larynx is the squamous cell carcinoma, which is more common in elderly males, smokers, and alcoholics. Patients may present with neck mass, dysphagia, stridor, and hemoptysis.

Supraglottic Carcinoma

Supraglottic carcinoma arises from the anterior compartment (epiglottis) and the posterolateral compartment (the aryepiglottic fold, the false vocal fold), the pre-epiglottic, and the paraglottic space. It metastasizes early with lymph nodes, due to the rich lymphatic network.

CLINICAL

Symptoms like hoarseness occur late, so patients present when the disease is at an advanced stage.

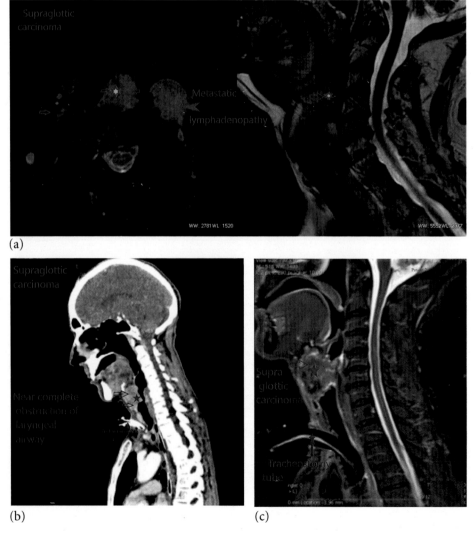

Figure 14.9 (a) MRI findings of supraglottic carcinoma, (b and c) imaging findings of supraglottic-glottic carcinomas.

IMAGING

- CT – asymmetry of the laryngeal side, with moderate enhancement on the involved side. Lymphadenopathy and tumor extension can be evaluated. Cartilage sclerosis may be noted.
- MRI – T1-hypointense and T2-hyperintense SI, with moderate heterogeneous enhancement and obliteration of paraglottic fat.

MANAGEMENT

Voice-conserving therapy may be conducted, unless tumor extends into the thyroid, arytenoid, and cricoid cartilages, the glottis or the pyriform fossa.

Glottic Carcinoma

It is a slow-growing and well-differentiated tumor, that arises from a true vocal cord.

CLINICAL

Hoarseness of voice. Rarely metastasizes *via* lymph nodes, due to poor lymphatic circulation of the glottis.

IMAGING

- CT – enhancing exophytic or infiltrative true vocal fold mass, which may extend to the anterior commissure, posterior commissure, or the supra- or subglottis
- MRI – T1-hypointense T2-hyperintense lesion with homogeneous enhancement

Subglottic Carcinoma

It arises from anywhere below the true vocal fold to the cricoid cartilage inferiorly.

CLINICAL

It metastasizes early but is diagnosed late, due to minimal symptoms in the initial stages. High propensity for nodal invasion, and thyroarytenoid involvement results in cord fixation.

IMAGING

- CT – well-defined, enhancing soft tissue density lesion in the subglottis.

MANAGEMENT

For glottic and infraglottic carcinomas, voice-conserving therapy is contraindicated, if the tumor extends into the thyroid cartilage, the anterior commissure, to involve the contralateral cord, the subglottic region and across the ventricle to the false cord.

Transglottic carcinoma involves more than one compartment when the site of origin is not clear.

Staging:

Tis – Carcinoma *in situ*
  T1 – Tumor limited to the region with unimpaired mobility
  T2 – Tumor expansion to adjacent areas without fixation
  T3 – Tumor limited to larynx with cord fixation, or exhibiting extensive infiltration
  T4 – Tumor with direct extension beyond the larynx
N – Node
  N0 – No regional lymph node involvement
  N1 – Involvement of movable ipsilateral regional lymph nodes
  N2 – Involvement of movable contralateral or bilateral regional lymph nodes
  N3 – Fixed regional nodes
M – Metastases
  M0 – No distant metastases
  M1 – Distant metastases noted

MANAGEMENT

Combined surgery and radiotherapy as per tumor staging. Small lesions may be treated with laser therapy or radiotherapy, whereas larger lesions may require total laryngectomy.

Submandibular Duct Calculi (Sialolithiasis)

These are calculi arising within the salivary glands and the associated ducts, with the submandibular gland hilum and Wharton's duct being the most common sites. As Wharton's duct is longer and has a narrower lumen in comparison to other salivary ducts, it is predisposed toward salivary stasis. Stagnant calcium-rich secretions eventually form stones. Sialadenitis, swelling, and inflammation of the gland may occur due to obstruction, infection, or autoimmune causes. It may progress to chronic form, resulting in atrophy of the gland.

CLINICAL

Colicky pain and swelling of the affected gland with meals.

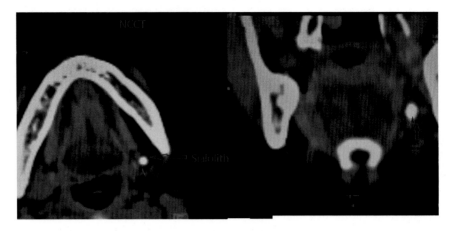

Figure 14.10 Imaging findings of sialolithiasis.

IMAGING

- NCCT – hyperdense calculi in the region of the duct and the gland
- CECT – evaluates the extent of inflammatory changes and adjacent stranding, though it may simulate a vessel filled with contrast material
- MRI reveals stones as signal voids and may mimic vessels
- MR sialography (heavily T2W sequence) – high sensitivity for ductal evaluation, including strictures, though it is contraindicated in acute sialadenitis

DDs

- Kussmaul disease, in which a mucus plug (instead of calculus) obstructs the duct and results in sialadenitis
- Hemangioma/phlebolith
- Vascular calcification

MANAGEMENT

- Conservative management, with NSAIDs for pain relief, antibiotics for infection, and moist warm heat with gland massage and sialogogues
- Sialolithotomy – extraction of the obstructing stones
- Endoscopic intracorporeal shear-wave lithotripsy (EISWL)

Pleomorphic Adenoma

A benign neoplasm of the salivary gland, common in the age group of 40–70 years, with a predominance of females.

CLINICAL

Painless, smooth, slow-growing mass.

IMAGING

The lesion is hypodense on NCCT, with heterogeneous enhancement on CECT.

- MRI – low SI on T1W, bright on T2W, and with intense enhancement

DDs

- Polymorphous low-grade adenocarcinoma.
- Mucoepidermoid carcinoma – most common primary malignant tumor of salivary glands
- Warthin's tumor (papillary cystadenoma lymphomatosum) – second-most common benign tumor of the parotid, with predominance of males, and involving older age groups of more than 50 years of age. It is usually bilateral and typically has well-circumscribed, smooth margins, and may have cystic components.

MANAGEMENT

Surgical excision to avoid recurrence.

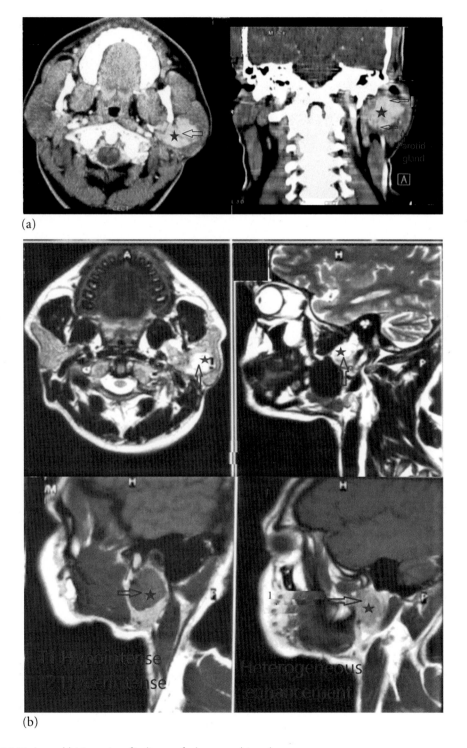

(a)

(b)

Figure 14.11 (a and b) Imaging findings of pleomorphic adenoma.

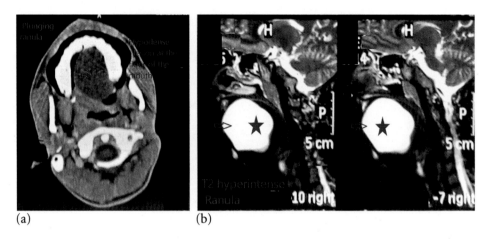

(a)   (b)

Figure 14.12 (a and b) Imaging findings of ranula.

Ranula

Benign, mucous-retentive cyst that occurs at the floor of the mouth, and results from obstruction of the sublingual gland or its duct. It can be simple (localized to the sublingual gland) or plunging type (extending to the submandibular space).

CLINICAL

Fluctuant, painless, slow-growing swelling.

IMAGING

- CT – thin-walled, non-enhancing, cystic lesion at the floor of the mouth. Attenuation may vary, depending on the proteinaceous contents of the lesion. Superimposed infection may cause thick, peripheral enhancement and adjacent fat/soft tissue stranding.
- MRI – Hypointense on T1WI, hyperintense on T2WI, with mild peripheral rim enhancement.

DDs

- Dermoids
- Epidermoid cysts
- Thyroglossal cysts
- Branchial cleft cysts

MANAGEMENT

Surgery.

SUGGESTED READING

Mittal, MK, Malik, A, Sureka, B, Thukral, BB. Cystic masses of neck: A pictorial review. *Indian Journal of Radiology and Imaging* 2012;22(4):334.

Osborn, AG, Salzman, KL, Jhaveri, MD, Barkovich, AJ. *Diagnostic Imaging: Brain.* Elsevier Health Sciences; 2015.

Peter Som, HC. *Head and Neck Imaging.* 5th ed. Mosby Inc., Elsevier; 2011.

15

Ear, Nose, and Paranasal Sinus

EAR

The temporal bone consists of five osseous components: the squamous, mastoid, petrous, tympanic, and styloid parts.

The external auditory canal (EAC), with lateral one-third cartilaginous and medial two-thirds bony composition, extends from the auricle to the tympanic membrane. The middle ear cavity is within the petrous portion of the temporal bone and consists of the tympanic cavity (containing the ossicles, namely the malleus, incus, and stapes) and the antrum. The mastoid antrum communicates with the epitympanum *via* aditus ad antrum. The middle ear also contains muscles (tensor tympani and stapedius), the round and oval windows, and the chorda tympani nerve. The inner ear consists of the osseous labyrinth (cochlea, vestibule, and the three semicircular canals, namely the superior, posterior, and lateral canals) and the membranous labyrinth (the cochlear duct, utricle, saccule, semicircular ducts, endolymphatic duct, and endolymphatic sac). The membranous labyrinth contains endolymph, surrounded by perilymph, and is enclosed within the bony labyrinth. The internal auditory canal (IAC) is located in the petrous bone and transmits facial and vestibulocochlear nerves along with the labyrinthine artery. The pars flaccida is the upper delicate part that is associated with Eustachian tube dysfunction and cholesteatoma. The pars tensa is larger and more robust, and associated with perforations.

Congenital Anomalies

EXTERNAL AND MIDDLE EAR

- Diffuse/focal stenosis
- Bony atresia of the external auditory meatus
- Malformed ossicles
- Absent short process of the malleus

INNER EAR

- Mondini's defect – abnormal cochlea, with 1.5 cochlear turns, enlarged vestibule, and vestibular aqueduct
- Michel's aplasia – complete labyrinthine aplasia
- Maldeveloped/hypoplastic semicircular canals
- Meniere's disease – congenital narrowing of the vestibular aqueduct (< 0.5 mm)
- Congenital dilatation of vestibular aqueduct (> 1.6–2.0 mm)
- Congenital enlargement of the cochlear duct; CSF leaks from oval window during stapedectomy (stapes gushers)

Pulsatile Tinnitus

NORMAL VASCULAR VARIANTS

- Aberrant ICA
- High-riding jugular bulb

PATHOLOGICAL CAUSES

- ICA dissection
- Atherosclerotic ICA
- Fibromuscular dysplasia (FMD)
- Petrous carotid aneurysm
- Transverse sinus thrombosis
- Intracranial hypertension
- Cerebral AVM
- Dural arteriovenous fistula
- Glomus tumor

CT evaluates whether the lesion is confined within the tympanic cavity or involves the jugular bulb.

MRI aids in assessing the internal jugular vein involvement.

NASAL CAVITY AND PARANASAL SINUSES

The nasal cavity is divided into two by a septum that is cartilaginous anteriorly and bony posteriorly. The nasal conchae/turbinates – superior, middle, and inferior – are thin, bony, curled bulges covered with mucosa. The conchae form the various nasal passages: the inferior, middle and superior nasal meatus.

The paranasal sinuses are air-filled spaces between the bones around the nasal cavity. Draining ostia connect four distinct sinuses with the nasal cavity. The anterior ethmoid cells, the frontal sinus, and maxillary sinus drain into the middle meatus. The posterior ethmoid cells and sphenoid sinus drain into the superior meatus. The nasolacrimal duct drains into the inferior nasal meatus.

Maxillary and ethmoid sinuses are aerated at birth. Sphenoid and frontal sinuses are pneumatized at around two and six years, respectively. Adult size may be reached by adolescence.

Maxillary Sinus

OSTEOMEATAL COMPLEX OR UNIT (OMC/OMU)

Best visualized in the coronal section, the OMC is the complex of structures that help in mucociliary and airflow drainage of the maxillary, anterior ethmoidal and frontal sinuses into the middle meatus. It consists of:

- The uncinate process – a hook-like process of the ethmoid bone in the lateral wall of the nose
- The maxillary sinus with ostia
- The ethmoid bulla (the posterior-most cells of the anterior ethmoid complex)
- The ethmoidal infundibulum
- The hiatus semilunaris – a semicircular opening in the lateral nasal wall

Ethmoid Sinus

The ethmoid sinus is divided into the anterior and posterior complex. Anterior cells drain into the middle meatus, whereas the posterior complex drains into the superior meatus.

Frontal Sinus

The frontal sinus is absent at birth. Pneumatization occurs between the first and twelfth years.

Sphenoid Sinus

The sphenoid sinus may contain multiple, vertical septations and drain through the spheno-ethmoid recess into the superior meatus.

Normal Anatomical Variations

Apart from causing recurrent sinusitis, the following anatomical variations are pivotal to report, to avoid complications during surgery.

- Nasal septal deviation.
- Pneumatization of crista galli.
- Hypoplastic frontal sinus.

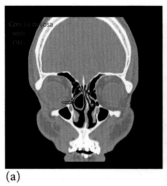
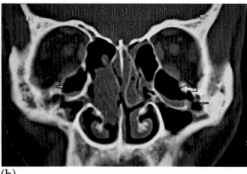

(a)   (b)

Figure 15.1 (a) Concha bullosa and deviated nasal septum, (b) Haller cells.

- Deep olfactory fossa – asymmetrical cribriform plate, that is developed more in the caudal direction. It may result in CSF leakage or meningitis, if it fractures during functional endoscopic sinus surgery (FESS).
- Agger nasi cells – the anterior-most cells of the anterior ethmoid complex, which may obstruct the frontal recess.
- Ethmoidal bulla – the posterior-most cells in the anterior ethmoidal complex.
- Haller cells – infraorbital ethmoid cells that may obstruct the ethmoidal infundibulum of the OMU.
- Onodi cells – posterior ethmoid cells that migrate to the anterior part of the sphenoid sinus. Its close relation to the optic nerve makes it clinically significant for reporting, prior to endoscopic sinus surgery.
- Supraorbital ethmoid cells are located posterolateral to the frontal sinus and may mimic multiple frontal sinuses on coronal CT.
- Paradoxical middle turbinate – abnormal curvature of the middle turbinate toward the midline.
- Concha bullosa – pneumatization of the middle turbinate, especially of its inferior. bulbous portion, which is one of the most frequently encountered anatomical variations.
- Pneumatization of the uncinate process.
- Pneumatization of the anterior clinoid process

Chronic Otitis Media with Mastoiditis

An inflammatory process of the middle ear and mastoid, which may occur due to Eustachian tube dysfunction or obstruction, viral or bacterial infection.

CLINICAL

Otalgia, otorrhea, headache, irritability, fever, hearing loss.

IMAGING

HRCT temporal bone:

- Soft tissue density/mucosal thickening in the middle ear cavity
- Thickened and bulging tympanic membrane, or perforation in chronic cases
- Hypopneumatization of mastoid with air-fluid level in the middle ear
- No bony erosion

MRI:

- Fluid signal in the middle ear cavity and mastoid antrum

DDs

- Cholesteatoma – a mass in the non-dependent areas, along with the bony destruction of ossicles and the lateral wall of the epitympanum
- Hemotympanum – a history of trauma and skull base fracture

MANAGEMENT

Antibiotics course.

ANCILLARY

- Coalescent mastoiditis leads to a loss of septae in mastoid cells and eventually results in cavity

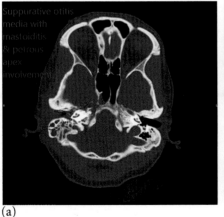 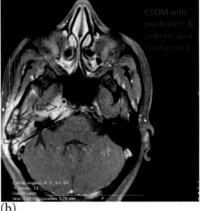

(a)   (b)

Figure 15.2 (a and b) Imaging findings of chronic otitis media with mastoiditis.

formation. It cannot be differentiated from early cholesteatoma, when there is no bony or ossicular chain erosive change.
- Petrous apicitis (Gradenigo's syndrome). Triad of:
  - Purulent otitis media
  - Pain along 6th nerve (abducens) distribution
  - Ipsilateral lateral rectus muscle palsy

Cholesteatoma

Most cholesteatomas are acquired, but some are congenital.

CLINICAL
Conductive hearing loss, otorrhea.

IMAGING
- CT – sharply marginated, expansile, soft tissue mass in the non-dependent location, with retraction of the tympanic membrane and blunting of the scutum. Large cholesteatomas can erode the auditory ossicles and the walls of the antrum and extend into the middle cranial fossa. The most affected structures are:
  - Auditory ossicles
  - Wall of the lateral semicircular canal
  - Lateral epitympanic wall (the scutum)
- CECT – non-enhancing or ring-like enhancement, with absence of central contrast enhancement, especially in larger lesions
- MRI – T1-hypointense, T2-hyperintense
- DWI – restricted diffusion

Two patterns of spread:

- *Pars flaccida cholesteatoma (Attic type)*

The lesion initiates anterosuperiorly in Prussak's space (the area just below the scutum), and then extends laterally toward the ossicular chain and into the epitympanum.
- *Pars tensa cholesteatoma (Sinus type)*

The cholesteatoma begins posterosuperiorly, then extends posteriorly toward the facial recess and the tympanic sinus, and medially toward the ossicular chain.

DDs (LOCATION-SPECIFIC)
Middle Ear Cholesteatoma
- Cholesterol granulomas
- Paragangliomas
- Facial nerve schwannoma – enlarged facial nerve canal and geniculate fossa, with a heterogeneously enhancing mass along the tympanic segment of the facial nerve
- Facial nerve hemangioma – enlarged facial nerve canal and geniculate fossa with honeycomb type strongly enhancing lesion

External Auditory Canal (EAC) Cholesteatomas

Keratosis obturans – bilateral keratin plugs within the enlarged EAC, usually in young patients with sinusitis and bronchiectasis.

- Cerumen (ear wax) – fat attenuation with a rim of air.
- Necrotizing external otitis – common in elderly, immunocompromised patients (usually with diabetes) suffering with a *Pseudomonas aeruginosa* infection. Extensive bony erosions and strong contrast enhancement at the base of the skull.

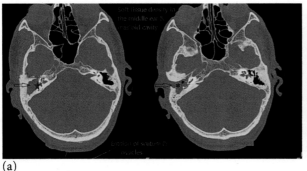
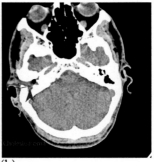

(a)　　　　　(b)

Figure 15.3 (a and b) CT findings of cholesteatoma.

- Squamous cell carcinoma of the EAC – frequent in elderly patients, and may sometimes be indistinguishable from a cholesteatoma.

MANAGEMENT

Surgery.

Cholesterol Granuloma

Chronic inflammatory reaction to repetitive episodes of bleeding in the middle ear, petrous apex, or mastoid air cells. It occurs mainly due to Eustachian tube dysfunction.

CLINICAL

Headache, hearing loss, vertigo.

IMAGING

CT:

- Expansile, cystic lesions, that cause smooth erosion of the petrous apex and thinning of the overlying bone. They can cause erosions of the internal auditory canal, otic capsule, carotid canal, and the jugular foramen.

MRI:

- High T1 signal due to cholesterol and methemoglobin
- High T2 signal centrally
- No central enhancement, but may show some faint peripheral enhancement
- No attenuation on FLAIR
- No suppression on fat saturation sequences

DWI:

- No restricted diffusion

DDs

- Cholesteatoma
- Effusions
- Thrombosed aneurysm
- Mucocele

MANAGEMENT

Surgery.

Antrochoanal Polyp

Solitary polyp that arises from the maxillary antrum, fills the sinus, and prolapses through the maxillary ostium to result in a characteristic dumbbell shape. It may extend into the nasal cavity and posteriorly to the choana, hence the term *antrochoanal polyp*. Because of its large stalk, it is susceptible to complications, such as torsion, strangulation, and even autoamputation and expulsion. It is often associated with allergies, nasal polyposis, cystic fibrosis, and chronic sinusitis.

CLINICAL

Unilateral obstruction, nasal congestion and discharge, breathing difficulty, and sinus infection.

IMAGING

CT:

- Well-defined hypodense mass, arising from the maxillary sinus, and leading to widening of the maxillary ostium, extending into the nasopharynx.

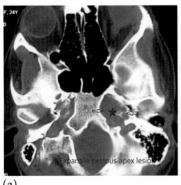
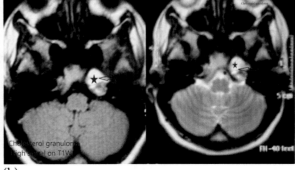

(a)   (b)

Figure 15.4 (a and b) Imaging findings of cholesterol granuloma.

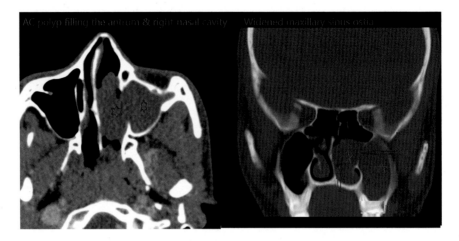

Figure 15.5 Imaging findings of antrochoanal polyp.

• Smooth expansion of the sinus without any bony destruction

MRI:

• Hypointense on T1WI and hyperintense on T2WI. Hyperintense on T1WI if the contents are proteinaceous
• Exhibits peripheral enhancement

DDs

• Inverted papilloma
• Nasoethmoidal encephalocele
• Maxillary sinus mucocele
• Acute sinusitis with edematous mucosa prolapsing from the maxillary antrum
• Sinonasal organized hematoma

MANAGEMENT

Functional endoscopic sinus surgery (FESS).

Frontoethmoidal Mucocele

Most common expansile mass of the paranasal sinus and is usually idiopathic or caused by obstruction of the ostium or inflammation, due to prior surgery or trauma of the sinuses. The frontal sinuses are the most frequently affected, followed by the ethmoid, maxillary, and sphenoid sinuses.

CLINICAL

Cystic swelling near the orbit, proptosis, orbital symptoms.

IMAGING

CT:

• Completely opacified, non-enhancing, and mucus-filled expanded sinus; homogeneous and isodense, relative to brain tissue
• Remodeled sinus walls may show thinning, erosion, and dehiscence
• Thin rim enhancement is seen in infected mucopyoceles

MRI appearance varies, depending on the contents of the mucocele, usually with T1 intermediate and T2 hyperintense signal intensity (SI).

Hyperattenuation on CT and low SI on T1W and T2W suggest inspissated secretions. More hydrated and proteinaceous secretions are associated with T1 and T2 hyperintensity, with isodense or hypodense appearance on CT.

DDs

• Mucous retention cyst – no bony expansion
• Tumor – diffusely enhancing
• Acute sinusitis – no bony expansion

MANAGEMENT

Endoscopic sinus surgery.

Osteomeatal Unit (OMU) Pattern Obstructive Sinusitis

Obstruction at the level of the middle meatus leads to inflammatory sinonasal disease within

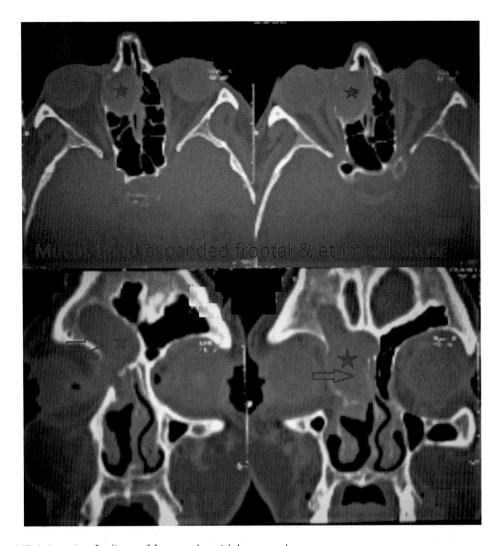

Figure 15.6 Imaging findings of frontoethmoidal mucocele.

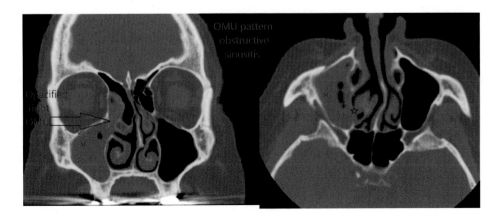

Figure 15.7 Imaging findings of OMU pattern obstructive sinusitis.

the ipsilateral maxillary, frontal, and anterior and middle ethmoid sinuses.

CLINICAL

Nasal obstruction, congestion postnasal drainage, headache, pain and swelling around the eyes, nose, and cheeks.

IMAGING

Acute Sinusitis

CT and MRI – mucosal thickening, submucosal edema, air-fluid levels, or sinus secretions, interspersed with air bubbles. Acute sinonasal secretions are mucoid in nature (–10 to 25 HU) and are typically hypointense on T1 and hyperintense on T2 sequences.

CHRONIC SINUSITIS

Mucosal thickening, sinus opacification, intrasinus calcifications, and sclerosis (reactive osteitis) of the bony walls of the sinus.

MANAGEMENT

FESS, if medical management fails.

Invasive Fungal Sinusitis

Usually unilateral, noted in immunocompromised or diabetic patients, and characterized by the presence of fungal hyphae within the mucosa, submucosa, bone, or blood vessels of the paranasal sinuses. It can be stratified into acute, chronic, or chronic granulomatous entities.

CLINICAL

Sinus pain, nasal discharge, low-grade fever, and epistaxis, recurrent infections, and orbital involvement (periorbital edema, ptosis, ophthalmoplegia, visual loss, or proptosis).

IMAGING

Acute Invasive Fungal Sinusitis

CT:

- Hypodense mucosal thickening or an area of soft tissue attenuation within the lumen of the involved paranasal sinus and nasal cavity
- Rapid and aggressive bone destruction of the sinus walls, with intracranial and intraorbital extension of the inflammation
- These fungi tend to extend along the vessels, and extension beyond the sinuses may occur with intact bony walls
- Intracranial extension of disease from the sphenoid sinus leads to cavernous sinus thrombosis and even carotid artery invasion, occlusion, or pseudoaneurysm, with resulting fatal cerebral infarct and hemorrhage

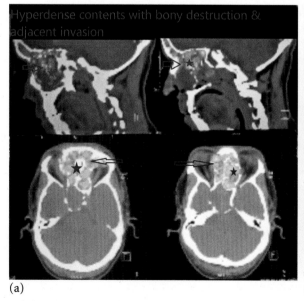

(a)

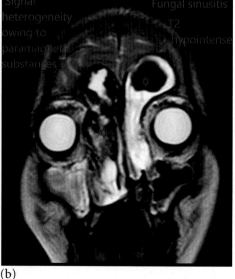

(b)

Figure 15.8 (a) CT findings of invasive fungal sinusitis, (b) MRI findings of fungal sinusitis.

MRI:

- Intracranial and intraorbital extension of the disease, along with obliteration of the periantral fat and adjacent fat stranding.
- Leptomeningeal enhancement, which may progress to cerebritis, granulomas, and cerebral abscess formation, suggests intracranial invasion.
- Intracranial granulomas appear iso- to hypointense on T1- and T2-weighted images, with minimal enhancement on contrast-enhanced images. The SI heterogeneity is due to the presence of paramagnetic substances such as iron and manganese.

Chronic Invasive Fungal Sinusitis (>12 weeks)

- NCCT – hyperdense mass in the sinus along with sclerosis and destruction of its bony walls, with extension into the adjacent structures, like the orbits, maxillary floor, and hard palate.
- MRI – hypointense signal on both T1 and T2WI

Chronic Invasive Granulomatous Sinusitis

Usually seen in immunocompetent patients, where imaging exhibits a large expansile mass hyperdense on the CT scan, hypointense on T2W, homogeneous contrast enhancement with osseous destruction and invasion of adjacent structures, like the orbits, nasal cavity, and skull base.

DDs

- Complicated acute and chronic viral or bacterial rhinosinusitis
- Wegener's granulomatosis (granulomatosis with polyangiitis)
- Sinonasal squamous cell carcinoma
- Sinonasal non-Hodgkin lymphoma

MANAGEMENT

Systemic antifungal (e.g., amphotericin B), followed by aggressive surgical debridement.

Treat diabetic ketoacidosis or neutropenia.

ANCILLARY

The noninvasive subtypes typically occur in immunocompetent individuals and include mycetoma and allergic fungal sinusitis, which are associated with a history of atopy, including allergic rhinitis or asthma. NCCT exhibits centrally hyperdense and peripherally hypodense material within multiple opacified and expanded sinuses.

Frontal (Ivory) Osteoma

Benign tumor most frequently diagnosed in middle age, with male predominance. It may be associated with Gardner's syndrome.

CLINICAL

Asymptomatic or headache, cerebrospinal fluid (CSF) fistula, meningitis, ptosis, diplopia, or pneumocephalus.

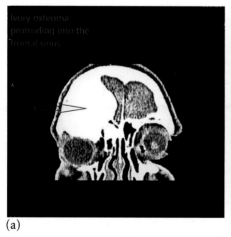

(a)

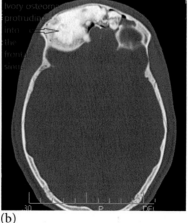

(b)

Figure 15.9 (a and b) Imaging findings of ivory osteoma.

IMAGING

- NCCT – well-circumscribed hyperdense lesion of bone density, arising from the calvaria and protruding into the sinus
- CECT – no enhancement
- MRI – non-enhancing heterogeneous low-to-intermediate SI lesion

DDs

- Fibrous dysplasia
- Meningioma
- Metaplastic dural ossification
- Osteogenic tumors like cemento-ossifying fibroma orosteoblastoma

MANAGEMENT

Symptomatic cases may need resection.

Juvenile Ossifying Fibroma

Rare, benign, rapidly growing, locally aggressive fibro-osseous lesion, with a tendency for recurrence. It is common in children under fifteen years of age.

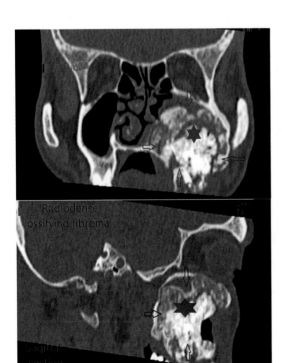

Figure 15.10 Imaging findings of ossifying fibroma.

CLINICAL

Facial swelling, nasal obstruction.

IMAGING

- CT – well-defined, radio-dense lesion, causing expansion of underlying bone, obliteration of maxillary sinus, and cortical thinning. Soft tissue components may enhance.

DDs

- Fibrous dysplasia
- Calcifying odontogenic tumor
- Osteosarcoma

MANAGEMENT

Surgery.

Esthesioneuroblastoma (ENB, Olfactory Neuroblastoma)

This uncommon malignant tumor of neural crest origin arises from neuroendocrine cells within the olfactory epithelium of the superior nasal cavity.

CLINICAL

Nasal obstruction, epistaxis, headache, anosmia.

IMAGING

- CT – homogeneously enhancing soft tissue density mass in the superior nasal cavity, which may extend into the ethmoid and maxillary sinuses, the orbit and the anterior cranial fossa
  - Intranasal and intracranial components, with relative narrowing at the level of cribriform plate, resulting in a characteristic dumbbell shape
- MRI – T1-hypointense and T2-hyperintense lesion with avid homogeneous enhancement
  - It may be associated with non-neoplastic peripheral cysts (due to the trapping of CSF within the clefts) at the tumor–brain interface (peritumoral cysts)
- DSA – prominent tumor blush, with arteriovenous shunting and persistent opacification
- MIBG (metaiodobenzylguanidine) avid on scintigraphy scan

DDs

- Olfactory neuroepithelioma
- Olfactory groove meningioma

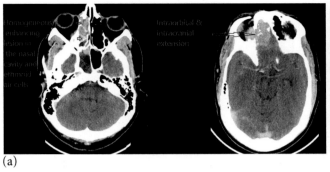
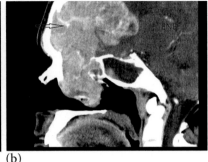

(a)   (b)

Figure 15.11 (a and b) CT findings of esthesioneuroblastoma.

- Sinonasal undifferentiated carcinoma
- Lymphoma
- Rhabdomyosarcoma

MANAGEMENT

Complete surgical resection with adjuvant chemotherapy/radiotherapy.

Nasopharyngeal Carcinoma

The most common nasopharyngeal tumor in adults, it has squamous cell origin and male predominance. Apart from its association with the Epstein-Barr virus (EBV), other predisposing factors include ingestion of nitrosamines (salt-preserved fish, foods), tobacco, and alcohol.

CLINICAL

Palpable cervical neck nodal mass, epistaxis, headache, conductive hearing loss, nasal obstruction, and discharge.

IMAGING

- CT – heterogeneously enhancing, paramedian nasopharyngeal mass that effaces the fossa of Rosenmuller and destroys adjacent osseous structures
  - Enhancing metastatic nodes with hypodense necrotic areas, which are delineated in the retropharyngeal and cervical region
  - Obstruction of pharyngeal orifice of the Eustachian tube results in serous otitis media
- MRI – T1-iso- to hypointense and T2-hyperintense lesion with heterogeneous enhancement

- FDG PET-CT – earlier detection of nodal metastasis, disease clearance, and simpler monitoring

DDs

- Prominent but normal adenoidal tissue is difficult to differentiate from small nasopharyngeal lesions, which are confined by the pharyngobasilar fascia
- Nasopharyngeal lymphoma
- Metastases
- Juvenile nasopharyngeal angiofibroma

MANAGEMENT

External-beam radiotherapy with chemotherapy.

Surgery may be considered for radiation-resistant tumors and in situations of local recurrence.

ANCILLARY

Any adult presenting with unexplained unilateral serous otitis media should be carefully examined to rule out NPC.

Juvenile Nasopharyngeal Angiofibroma

Benign, though aggressively vascular tumors of the nasopharynx, they occur almost exclusively in adolescent males. They arise in the sphenopalatine foramen area and extend into the nasopharynx and infratemporal fossa through the pterygopalatine fossa. The tumor is usually sessile, globular, and relatively hard.

CLINICAL

Life-threatening, with recurrent epistaxis, and chronic otomastoiditis, due to obstruction of the Eustachian tube.

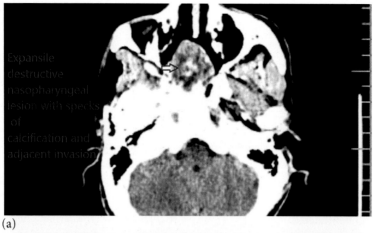

(a)

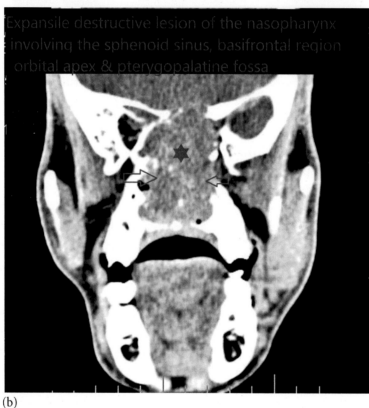

(b)

Figure 15.12 (a and b) Imaging findings of nasopharyngeal carcinoma.

IMAGING

- NCCT – soft tissue density lesion, arising from the sphenopalatine foramen on the lateral nasopharyngeal wall
  - It extends into the adjacent pterygopalatine fossa, resulting in widening of the fossa and anterior bowing of the posterior wall of the maxillary sinus
  - It may also extend intracranially and into the infratemporal fossa and sphenoid sinuses, resulting in the widening of the central skull base foramina and fissures
- CECT – intense enhancement of the lesion
- MRI – intermediate signal on T1 and hetero-geneous signal with flow voids on T2WI, with intense enhancement

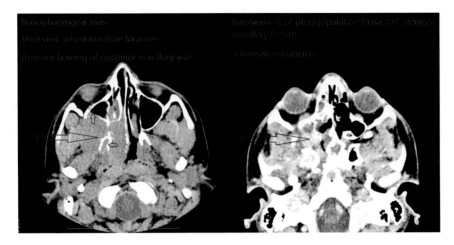

Figure 15.13 Imaging findings of juvenile nasopharyngeal angiofibroma.

- Angiography – dense homogeneous blush persisting into the venous phase
  - Feeding arteries include the internal maxillary artery and the ascending pharyngeal artery

This intensely vascular lesion should never be biopsied, and the diagnosis should be made on the basis of angiography.

DDs

- Angiomatous polyp
- Nasopharyngeal carcinoma
- Esthesioneuroblastoma

MANAGEMENT

Complete surgical excision with preoperative embolization.

Ameloblastoma (Adamantinoma of the Jaw)

Locally aggressive, slow-growing, benign, epithelial, odontogenic tumor, near the angle of the mandible (posterior mandible in the third molar region, with an impacted tooth).

CLINICAL

Painless bony deformity.

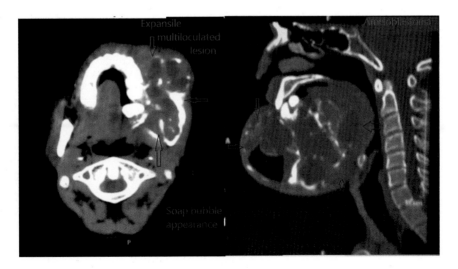

Figure 15.14 Imaging findings of ameloblastoma.

IMAGING

- CT – expansile, well-marginated uni-/multi-loculated lesion with "soap bubble" appearance and without calcifications
  - Resorption of adjacent teeth
  - Adjacent cortical erosion may extend the lesion into the surrounding oral mucosa
- MRI – thick-walled, mixed solid-cystic lesion, with enhancing solid components

DDs

- Odontogenic keratocyst, usually unilocular, less expansile with thin, poorly enhancing walls
- Dentigerous cyst
- Odontogenic myxoma
- Giant cell reparative granuloma
- Calcifying epithelial odontogenic tumor (Pindborg tumor)

MANAGEMENT

Surgical resection.

Dentigerous Cyst (Follicular Cyst)

A slow-growing, non-inflammatory, developmental cyst.

CLINICAL

Painless lesion.

IMAGING

- CT – unilocular, lucent lesion, associated with the crown of an impacted/unerupted tooth,

with mandibular and maxillary third molars being the most common sites
- MRI – non-enhancing lesion, hypointense on T1WI and hyperintense on T2WI

DDs

- Radicular cysts are the most common; associated with tooth infection, caries
- Odontogenic keratocyst – T1-hyperintense, due to keratin content
- Aneurysmal bone cyst

MANAGEMENT

Removal of cyst along with unerupted tooth.

ANCILLARY

Multiple cysts are associated with basal cell nevus syndrome.

Thornwaldt Cyst

Benign, developmental posterior nasopharyngeal notochord remnant.

CLINICAL

Asymptomatic or intermittent halitosis, unpleasant taste, and occipital headache if the cyst gets infected.

IMAGING

- CT – well-circumscribed, thin-walled, midline hypodense cystic lesion, located in the posterior nasopharyngeal wall, between and anterior to the longus colli muscles

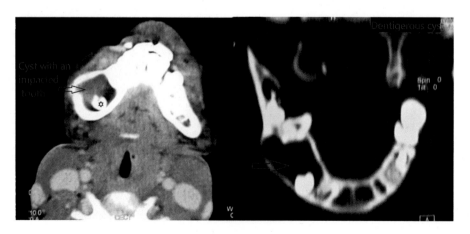

Figure 15.15 Imaging findings of a dentigerous cyst.

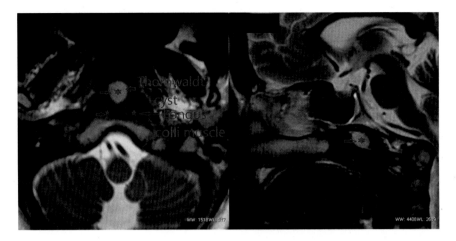

Figure 15.16 Imaging findings of a Thornwaldt cyst.

- Faint rim enhancement may be seen
- MRI – T1- iso- to hyperintense and T2 hyper- to hypointense lesion, depending on the protein content of the lesion

DDs

- Retention cyst
- Vallecular cyst (paramedian location)
- Neurenteric cysts
- Choanal polyp
- Adenoidal inflammation

MANAGEMENT

Usually, no treatment is required. If necessary, marsupialization of the cyst can be carried out, along with antibiotic therapy.

Rhinolith (Nasal Calculi)

Chronic inflammatory response to foreign body or trauma in the nasal cavity. Common in children and mentally impaired adults. Maybe iatrogenic, due to old nasal packing.

CLINICAL

Unilateral, purulent nasal discharge, nasal obstruction.

IMAGING

- CT – calcified lesion in the nasal cavity
  - Associated mucosal thickening

DDs

Osteoma.

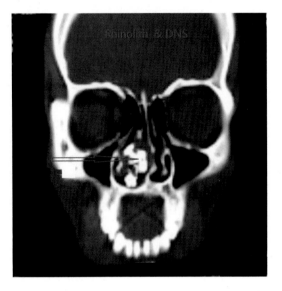

Figure 15.17 Rhinolith.

MANAGEMENT

Endoscopic removal.

SUGGESTED READING

Adam, A. *Grainger & Allison's Diagnostic Radiology: A Textbook of Medical Imaging.* Churchill Livingstone; 2008.

Nadgir, R, Yousem, DM. *Neuroradiology: The Requisites.* 4th ed. Philadelphia: Elsevier; 2017.

Peter Som, HC. *Head and Neck Imaging.* 5th ed. Mosby Inc., Elsevier; 2011.

Reddy, UD, Dev, B. Pictorial essay: Anatomical variations of paranasal sinuses on multidetector computed tomography—How does it help FESS surgeons? *Indian Journal of Radiology & Imaging* 2012;22(4):317–324.

16

Miscellaneous

EPILEPSY

Abnormal excessive neuronal activation in the gray matter of the cerebral cortex.

TYPES

Focal (Partial)

Focal epilepsy can be simple (patient is conscious) or complex (impaired consciousness) and is usually initiated in the temporal lobe.

Generalized

Generalized epilepsy occurs where the focal seizure transmits to other parts of the brain. The patient is unconscious, and it can include absence seizures, myoclonic, tonic, clonic, tonic-clonic, or atonic types of seizures.

ETIOLOGY

- *Hippocampal sclerosis*
  Neuronal loss and gliosis, maximal in hippocampal subfields CA1 and CA4.
- *Neoplasms* (Chapter 4)
  Slow-growing, benign, cortical-based, located in the temporal lobe, and associated with developmental malformations.
  a) Pleomorphic xanthoastrocytoma (PXA)
  b) Dysembryoblastic neuroepithelial tumor
  c) Gangliogliomas – small cystic lesion with an enhancing nodule
  d) Hypothalamic hamartoma
- *Gray matter heterotopia*
- *Vascular lesions (cavernomas and AVMs)*
- *Malformations of cortical development*

Focal cortical dysplasia is a non-enhancing focal area of abnormal brain development, presenting as subcortical white matter hyperintensities and blurred gray–white matter interface. Sometimes, the hyperintensity extends from the subcortical area to the ventricular margin ("transmantle" sign).
- *Phakomatoses*
- *Rasmussen's encephalitis*
  Progressive hemiatrophy, leading to intractable seizures.
- *Ulegyria/post-traumatic injury*
  Ulegyria is a cortical scar due to ischemic injury in full-term infants. Minimal perfusion at the deeper portions of the gyri leads to its shrinkage and atrophy in comparison with the apical part of the gyri, giving it a characteristic mushroom shape. Other types of cortical and glial scars may result from infective or traumatic injury.
- Drugs, dehydration, lack of sleep, fever without any irritant focus in the brain may cause seizures.

EPILEPSY PROTOCOL

- CT – calcifications
- T1WI – cortical thickness, gray–white matter interface, or any heterotopias
- FLAIR and T2WI – subtle cortical and subcortical hyperintensities
- T2 or SWI – hemoglobin breakdown products (post-trauma, cavernomas)

Calcifications (tuberous sclerosis, Sturge-Weber syndrome, cavernomas, and gangliogliomas).

- MRS – decreased concentration of N-acetyl aspartate (NAA).

Mesial Temporal Sclerosis (MTS) (Hippocampal Sclerosis)

Usually, it is unilateral but, in a few cases, it can be bilateral.

CLINICAL

Intractable seizures are refractory to medical management.

IMAGING

- Coronal high-resolution T2WI/FLAIR is the best modality by which to diagnose MTS. Axial sections might miss the pathology. It is challenging to compare the contralateral hippocampus and hence to diagnose bilateral MTS. Asymmetry and abnormal signal within the atrophied hippocampus is the hallmark of MTS:
  - Volume loss due to hippocampal atrophy
  - High signal intensity on T2 and FLAIR images is suggestive of gliosis
  - Secondary dilatation of the temporal horn of the lateral ventricle
  - Blurred parahippocampal gray–white matter differentiation
- Quantitative three-dimensional volume measurements of each hippocampus – subtle hippocampal atrophy.
- T2 relaxometry – hippocampal sclerosis.
- MRS – reduced N-acetyl aspartate (NAA) and myo-inositol (MI) levels in the ipsilateral temporal lobe and postictal increase in lipid-lactate.
- MR perfusion – increases in peri-ictal phase and decreases in the interictal phase.

DDs

Unilateral dilatation of the hippocampal or choroidal fissure of the temporal horn – common normal variant and does not necessarily indicate hippocampal atrophy.

MANAGEMENT

Anti-epileptics initially. Temporal lobectomy or selective amygdalohippocampectomy (refractory conditions).

Empty Sella

Variant where the pituitary gland is compressed against the sellar wall, arachnoid space, or where CSF herniates into the pituitary fossa through the deficient diaphragma sella.

- May be primary (idiopathic) or secondary (owing to a known cause, like previous surgery, trauma, tumors, hemorrhage, etc.)
- Particularly common in obese and hypertensive middle-aged females

CLINICAL

Asymptomatic, headache, and visual disturbances.

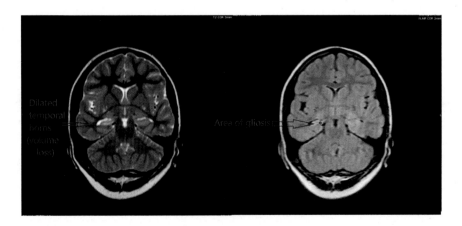

Figure 16.1 MRI findings of mesial temporal sclerosis.

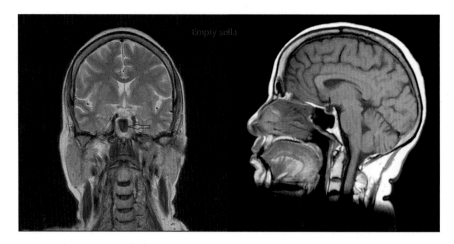

Figure 16.2 Imaging findings of empty sella.

IMAGING

CT and MRI:

- A variable-sized, CSF-filled fossa through which an infundibulum may be seen traversing ("infundibulum" sign)
- Small, shrunken pituitary gland

It is also associated with idiopathic intracranial hypertension (IIH), also known as pseudotumor cerebri, which results in raised intracranial pressure without an intracranial mass lesion or hydrocephalus. The imaging findings include:

- Flattened posterior sclera
- Distended peri-optic nerve sheath (high SI)
- Tortuous optic nerve sheath complex

DDs

- Arachnoid cyst – mass effect on infundibulum and perceptible cyst wall
- Rathke's cleft cyst – small T2-hypointense dot ("dot" sign)

MANAGEMENT

No treatment is required.

AI IN RADIOLOGY

Artificial intelligence (AI) is a branch of computer science that is focused on making intelligent machines capable of mimicking human cognitive functions. First developed as an academic discipline in the 1950s, AI has, in recent years, found practical applications in a wide range of fields. Medicine is a field which is particularly set to be revolutionized by the upcoming waves of AI. The areas of medicine that involve diagnosis based on images, like neuroradiology, the topic of this book, will see even more significant changes as data availability increases and better algorithms are developed, or existing algorithms are applied in innovative ways. Image-processing algorithms, like SIFT, Principal Component Analysis, SURF, and others, offer promising future areas of research, especially when combined with other techniques. Currently, Convolutional Neural Networks (CNNs) are the most popular classification algorithms for images, with various architectures suited to different needs. A variety of algorithms is essential because, using AI to identify features in images and to diagnose medical conditions, will be a significant area of research and application going forward. With these tools and capabilities, AI is poised to bring drastic changes to neuroradiology.

What AI Can Do

AI has the potential to help radiologists battle their increasing workloads, especially in developing countries, where there is often a shortage of trained radiologists, and, thus, the existing ones are overworked. In these cases, AI-based diagnostic algorithms can offer a useful second opinion that either supports a doctor's decision or contradicts it, in which case another radiologist can review the diagnosis. Integrating the algorithm into the diagnostic process will reduce workloads and increase accuracy by adding an AI system that can provide valuable feedback collected from a dataset of tens of thousands of previous diagnoses. In fact, a Stanford-led study found that their algorithm CheXNeXt matched radiologists' accuracy in detecting 10 out of the 14 diseases tested, and even outperformed them on one disease, showing that the technology had promise as a valid second opinion.

There are other benefits as well. Some algorithms, like the aforementioned Principal Component Analysis (PCA), can be used to extract quantitative features from images, allowing radiologists to discover helpful new patterns that can be used to draw correlations and find previously unknown patterns among the disease scans. This area, called radiomics, involves sifting through large amounts of data of all kinds, to discover potentially actionable information that can be applied productively in the future. In a way, the AI algorithm acts as a radiologist's assistant, screening gargantuan amounts of patients' data to find patterns that can help in making future diagnoses.

Another benefit of AI is the potential reduction in acquisition time, which the NYU School of Medicine and Facebook are jointly researching. Currently, MRI scans take 20–60 minutes to complete, which is much more than the time taken for CT and X-rays scans. The team proposes training a neural network to recognize the underlying details of MRI scans; the system then uses this training to fill in missing information in the 'fast scans,' which will have less exposure time. The reduced time will increase the quality of experience for patients, while also improving image quality, because less time equals less patient movement. Wait time can also be reduced, allowing more patients to access MRI services, which is especially important in developing and underdeveloped countries.

Through advances like these, AI can aid radiologists and make various processes more efficient, accurate, and even enjoyable, while also providing new insights. However, it's not all sunshine and roses.

What AI Cannot Do

Despite the various ominous predictions, that AI will replace radiologists, such claims do not represent the reality of the field of radiology, since there are numerous currently-unresolved problems with AI systems.

Most of the technology is not yet ready, as most current AI systems cannot handle the peculiarities of the real world and thus are unable to perform as promised in hospital settings. Even if this technology vastly improves in the future, trained radiologists are still needed as they can connect all the details about a patient's history to make better decisions. They use their years of training to determine disease progression from past images, while also working with other healthcare teams and departments to make crucial medical decisions.

Furthermore, there are various ethical and legal concerns. Due to the vast amounts of data needed to train AI systems – data that will have to be collected from living human patients – strict ethical standards need to be put in place to ensure fair use and to provide privacy protection of personal data. Cybersecurity must also be increased to protect data from falling into the hands of hackers, who could use it for all sorts of malicious purposes. There is also the major question of legal responsibility. Governments must determine where liability falls in the case of misdiagnosis or medical negligence as a result of AI.

Ultimately, various issues need to be overcome before the widespread proliferation of AI occurs in radiology, and in medicine in general, and even then, AI will be able to only augment radiologists' workflow, not replace them entirely.

SUGGESTED READING

Sai Balasubramanian, JD. Artificial intelligence is not ready for the intricacies of radiology. *Forbes*, 2020 February 3.

Tang, A, Tam, R, Cadrin-Chênevert, A, Guest, W, Chong, J, Barfett, J, et al. Canadian association of radiologists white paper on artificial intelligence in radiology. *Canadian Association of Radiologists Journal* 2018;69(2):120–135.

Radiology Business. What has artificial intelligence done for radiology lately? 2019. Available at: https://www.radiologybusiness.com/topics/ai-machine-learning/what-has-artificial-intelligence-done-radiology-lately (accessed February 28, 2020).

Index